DAY TREATMENT FOR CHILDREN WITH EMOTIONAL DISORDERS

Volume 2
Models Across the Country

DAY TREATMENT FOR CHILDREN WITH EMOTIONAL DISORDERS
Volume 2
Models Across the Country

Edited by

Gordon K. Farley
and
Sara Goodman Zimet

University of Colorado Health Sciences Center
Denver, Colorado

PLENUM PRESS • NEW YORK AND LONDON

Library of Congress Cataloging in Publication Data

(Revised for vol. 2)

Day treatment for children with emotional disorders.

Includes bibliographical references and index.
Contents: v. 1. A model in action—v. 2. Models across the country.
1. Psychiatric day treatment for children—United States. I. Zimet, Sara Goodman. II.
Farley, Gordon K. [DNLM: 1. Affective Disorders—in infancy & childhood. 2. Affective
Disorders—therapy. 3. Day Care—in infancy & childhood. 4. Day Care—organization &
administration. WS 350.6 / D275]
RJ504.53.D38   1991   618.92'89   91-2086
ISBN 0-306-43744-9 (v. 2)

ISBN 0-306-43744-9

© 1991 Plenum Press, New York
A Division of Plenum Publishing Corporation
233 Spring Street, New York, N.Y. 10013

Printed in the United States of America

Dedicated to my wife, Kiki;
my sons, Steven and David;
my mother, Neva; my brothers, Curtis and Robert;
and my sister, Patricia.

—GKF

Dedicated to my husband, Carl;
and to my children, Greg, Andy,
Lynne, and Flo.

—SGZ

Contributors

Gaston E. Blom, South Shore Mental Health Center, 77 Parking Way, Quincy, Massachusetts 02169

Robert Catenaccio, 512 Mamaroneck Avenue, White Plains, New York 10605

Mark Finn, Psychology Department, North Central Bronx Hospital, 342 Kossuth Avenue, Bronx, New York 10454

Stewart Gabel, Department of Psychiatry, Cornell University Medical College, New York Hospital–Cornell Medical Center, Westchester Division, White Plains, New York 10605

Victor Hornbein, 266 Jackson Street, Denver, Colorado 80206

Joan A. Jordan, Exceptional Students Division, Georgia Department of Education, 1952 Twin Towers East, Atlanta, Georgia 30334

Laurel J. Kiser, Day Treatment Program, University of Tennessee, Memphis, Tennessee 38105

Robert D. Lyman, Department of Psychology, University of Alabama, Tuscaloosa, Alabama 35487

C. Janet Newman, Department of Psychiatry, College of Medicine, University of Cincinnati, Cincinnati, Ohio 45267

Steven Prentice-Dunn, Department of Psychology, University of Alabama, Tuscaloosa, Alabama 35487

David B. Pruitt, Day Treatment Program, University of Tennessee, Memphis, Tennessee 38105

Ellie F. Sternquist, P.O. Box 514, 3419 Harborview Drive, Gig Harbor, Washington 98335

William W. Swan, Department of Educational Administration, University of Georgia, Athens, Georgia 30602

Mary M. Wood, 575 Milledge Circle, Athens, Georgia 30606

Sara Goodman Zimet, the Day Care Center, Department of Psychiatry, University of Colorado Health Sciences Center, Denver, Colorado 80262

Preface

The life span of day treatment for children in the United States is relatively short, covering a period of about 50 years. Although the first 20 years saw little growth in the number of centers operating around the country, the concept of day treatment was recognized by the Joint Commission on Mental Illness and Health in 1961 as the most significant treatment innovation of this century. Enthusiasm for this treatment modality gained impetus from growing dissatisfaction among many mental health care providers who had no choice but to place children in a highly restrictive hospital environment. Day treatment did not carry the stigma associated with inpatient placement. The children could now remain with their own families and within their own communities. The parents could be actively included in their child's treatment. This new modality avoided the short- and long-term negative effects of institutionalization, and there was a favorable cost discrepancy between day and inpatient mental health services. In more recent years, there has been growing evidence of the efficacy of day treatment as an intensive therapeutic environment for children and their parents. Despite these advantages, day treatment has continued to be underutilized in favor of inpatient treatment by both the psychiatric community and third-party payers. Only recently is it being acknowledged by some insurers as a therapeutically sound and financially advantageous alternative to inpatient services. Consequently, it is showing signs of intense growth nationally.

In order to meet the demands for day treatment mental health services, we need answers to questions regarding the "nuts and bolts" of starting up a center; we need to review the wisdom gained by centers that have been operating programs successfully; we need to consider the range of choices in theoretical models and in treatment components. It is the purpose of the two volumes comprising *Day*

Treatment for Children with Emotional Disorders to present this information to both the novice and experienced practitioner and to the academician.

In Volume 2, *Models Across the Country,* we have focused on both practical and theoretical issues in three parts. The first part consists of three chapters dealing with issues about starting up day treatment services. The second part includes six chapters, each describing a day treatment program from a different theoretical perspective. The final part, the Appendix, provides the reader with a comprehensive annotated bibliography of publications on day treatment for children with emotional disorders.

In Volume 1, *A Model in Action,* we have examined the salient features of an actual program that has been operating since 1962—the Day Care Center. It is located within the Division of Child Psychiatry, Department of Psychiatry, of the University of Colorado Health Sciences Center. The primary focus of the chapters in this volume is the personal and practical issues of operating this program. We have presented the reader with a clinical case study of our program by describing its various components and the forces from within and from without that bear upon its day-to-day functioning. The volume is organized around four parts. The first part is introductory. The second part focuses on our clinical and educational programs and includes nine chapters of detailed descriptions. Administrative issues are examined in two chapters in the third part. The three chapters in our concluding part concentrate on our research and program evaluation efforts.

To those of our readers who are interested in learning about day treatment in Western Europe, we would like to refer them to two issues of the *International Journal of Partial Hospitalization* that were edited by us (1988, Volume 5, Numbers 1 and 2). They include descriptions of programs in England, France, The Netherlands, Norway, Sweden, Switzerland, and Germany. Five of the chapters are written by mental health professionals in those countries and six by Sara Goodman Zimet as a result of a fellowship she received from the World Rehabilitation Fund's International Exchange of Experts and Information in Rehabilitation. The fellowship was supported (in part) from a grant from the National Institute of Disability and Rehabilitation Research, U.S. Department of Education, Washington, DC 20201, Grant No. G008435012. Commentaries on each of the descriptions were made by Gordon K. Farley, who has been director of the Day Care Center for over 17 years.

In the process of preparing these volumes, we realized that there are many terms in current use that describe the day treatment modality, such as *day hospital, partial hospital, psychoeducational treatment center, psychiatric day treatment,* and so forth. Although our own center is located within a university health sciences center, we decided to use *day treatment* as the generic term that would apply to hospital-affiliated and nonaffiliated treatment programs. In making this choice, we have attempted to identify this treatment modality as existing within the child's and parents' community rather than within an institution separated from that community.

We would like to thank the children at the Day Care Center who contributed their illustrations to the two volumes comprising *Day Treatment for Children with Emotional Disorders.* These illustrations were done during their routine work with their art teacher (and head teacher), Ralph Imhoff. We are also indebted to Richard Simons, professor of psychiatry at the University of Colorado Health Sciences Center, for his helpful suggestions regarding our editorial role.

GORDON K. FARLEY
SARA GOODMAN ZIMET

Denver, Colorado

Contents

I

How to Start a Treatment Program

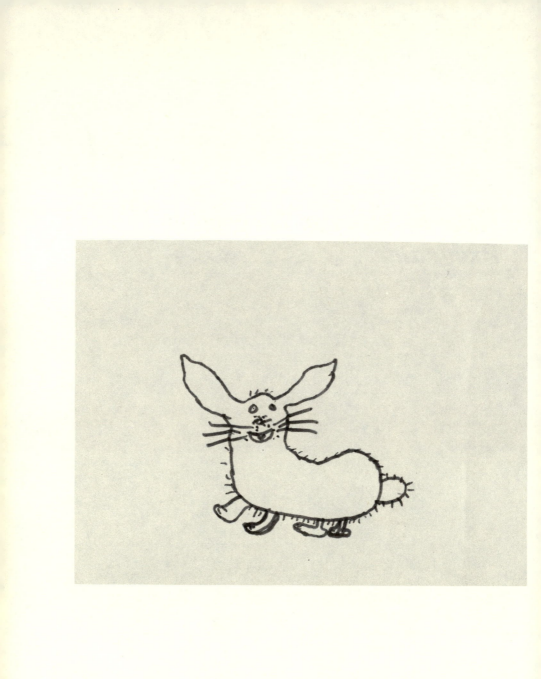

We have been providing day treatment for children for nearly 30 years and have accumulated an extensive list of questions that are commonly asked of us. One of the most common is, "How do you start up a program?" Another is, "What were the major problems during your early years, and how did you solve or attempt to solve them?" These obviously represent some of the most pressing questions around the organization and beginning of a day treatment center.

As the reader will see, many different patterns of start-up and financing are possible. The first chapter, by William Swan, a clinical psychologist, Mary Wood, a professor of special education, and Joan Jordan, an administrator in the State of Georgia Department of Education, contains information on building a unique statewide program for mental health services for children. Each of these authors was important in beginning this innovative model program. An important part of this comprehensive statewide service, in fact its cornerstone, is day psychiatric treatment. This is, perhaps, the only statewide model in the United States that makes day treatment an integral part.

The second chapter, by Laurel Kiser and David Pruitt, respectively, a clinical psychologist with a master's degree in business administration, and a child psychiatrist, recounts the experience of setting up a day treatment program in a university health sciences center and details the considerable assets and also some of the liabilities of such a venture. Each of them had an important role in starting up this unique program.

The third chapter investigates architectural considerations in the construction of a building that was specifically planned for a day treatment center for children. It is a rare opportunity to plan a day treatment center from the ground up, and in this chapter by Victor Hornbein, we are privy to the private musings of a thoughtful and sensitive architect whose primary concern is designing the best treatment setting possible.

1

Building a Statewide Program of Mental Health and Special Education Services for Children and Youth

WILLIAM W. SWAN, MARY M. WOOD,
and JOAN A. JORDAN

INTRODUCTION

Providing effective and comprehensive mental health services has been recognized as a major goal for the health care system for many decades. Yet serious obstacles persist as deterrents to accomplishment of adequate nationwide mental health services. Large case loads, undertrained staff, insufficient time for treatment, lack of comprehensive interdisciplinary staffing, astronomical costs for hospitalization, and shortages of alternative, supportive living environments are some of the major problems embedded in the current mental health delivery system (Hunter & Riger, 1986). In addition, though there may be pockets of effective mental health programs in some urban communities, critical shortages of programs and skilled personnel exist in rural communities.

WILLIAM W. SWAN • Department of Educational Administration, University of Georgia, Athens, Georgia 30602.   **MARY M. WOOD** • 575 Milledge Circle, Athens, Georgia 30606.   **JOAN A. JORDAN** • Exceptional Students Division, Georgia Department of Education, 1952 Twin Towers East, Atlanta, Georgia 30334.

When mental health services for children and youth are reviewed, the situation is worse. Compulsory education requires that the educational system maintain emotionally disturbed students, willing or not, in the schools. Public Law 94-142 (1975) as amended by Public Laws 98-199 (1983) and 99-457 (1986) further defines the rights of the handicapped, including those with serious emotional disturbances (SED), to an adequate and appropriate education in the least restrictive environment. With this legislative mandate at the national level and similar requirements for the states, the nation's schools have become the primary site for services to SED children and youth. Yet the schools generally have failed to provide programs of the type and quality needed by these students. A conservative estimate by Apter (1982) suggests that three-quarters of a million seriously disturbed children are not receiving special education.

Special education programs provided to students with serious emotional and behavioral problems typically are staffed by personnel who lack clinical training. Yet these teachers spend sustained periods of time daily attempting to provide individualized educational programs often based on assessment data as limited as IQ and achievement test results (Blom, Lininger, & Charlesworth, 1987; Zabel, Peterson, Smith, & White, 1982). Mental health specialists such as clinical social workers, clinical psychologists, psychiatrists, and those specializing in art, music, occupational and recreational therapies are seldom available. Walker (1982) summarizes the difficulties facing this field and the resulting gradual, but significant, national failure on the part of the schools to affect positive changes with SED students.

> Because of competing models of human behavior, psychological assessment, and therapy, and a reliance upon medically-based clinically-oriented definitional and classification systems that often have only limited applicability to the school setting, the field has exhibited a kind of paralysis and ambivalence regarding its legitimate domains of activity. (p. 52)

This failure with SED students by the educational system is cause for grave concern among mental health professionals and educators. Community mental health services have the personnel with experience and training to deliver effective mental health programs. Yet the typical mental health clinic environment is seldom the best location to deliver the service. Successful experiences in schools, families, and neighborhoods can produce healthy social and psychological changes (Gottlieb, 1981). Yet such changes usually do not occur without careful planning and skilled interdisciplinary service delivery. Many educators, mental health professionals, and child development specialists are advocating a reexamination of service delivery systems for SED children and youth, seeking ways to accomplish desired mental health gains within school settings.

THE GEORGIA PSYCHOEDUCATIONAL PROGRAM NETWORK

One unique statewide system of community-based, comprehensive mental health and special education services that has successfully addressed many of these problems is the Georgia Psychoeducational Program Network (Jordan, 1985). The network is a valuable model for program and policy planners to examine because of its successful 17-year history of interagency collaboration and service delivery at the state and local levels. Fully funded by the state, the network extends combined mental health and special education services to every school district in the state. Through the network, each of the state's 186 local county and city school districts and between 9,000 and 10,000 SED children and youth (birth to age 18) and their families receive comprehensive community-based psychoeducational services annually. This number represents about one-half of 1% of the total population (birth to age 18) in the state. Services are provided by 1,130 psychoeducational personnel statewide at a current cost of $2,298 per SED student annually (Georgia Department of Education, 1985; Jordan, 1985).

The network has a standard statewide program evaluation and documentation system for the 24 locally operated units that comprise the network (Georgia Department of Education, 1988b). Each of these local units operates in a designated multicounty geographic area and is a link in the flow of services between the local school system it serves, the area community health centers, and the regional mental hospitals. Each unit has a central location within its highest density population area and also provides services to several outposts in less densely populated rural areas within its geographic area. In this way, comprehensive coordinated mental health and special education services are available to each of the 186 local school districts and every SED child in Georgia.

The units that comprise the network are coordinated at the state level by the Georgia Department of Education using the State Advisory Panel and the Quality Basic Education Act Coordinating Council, including members representing mental health services, family and children services, vocational education, rehabilitation services, the Department of Corrections and Juvenile services. This interagency coordination provides interagency dialogue and planning. The network concept enhances interdisciplinary and interagency collaboration among personnel at the local and state levels and across agencies. Perhaps most notable is the sustained support the network has received from the state's legislators, governors, school superintendents, citizen groups, educators, and parents (Platt, 1973).

THE DEVELOPMENT OF THE NETWORK

To address the need for comprehensive and coordinated services to SED children and youth, the first community mental health and school-based service delivery prototype was initiated in Georgia in 1970 (Platt, 1973; Wood, 1972a,b,c; Wood & Fendley, 1971; Wood, Quirk, & Swan, 1971). This early prototype, the Rutland Center, was replicated and expanded systematically for 13 years to form the Georgia Psychoeducational Network (Pettit, 1974). Seventeen years later, the network continues to be the major service delivery vehicle in the state for mental health and special education services to SED children, youth, and their families (Georgia Department of Education, 1982, 1985; Swan, 1987; Swan, Purvis, & Wood, 1986). The phases of Network development are described next.

Public and Professional Awareness about Statewide Needs

Before the original network prototype was developed, it was noted that there were agencies and services available to SED children and youth in various locations in the state. Yet the services were neither comprehensive nor coordinated and were not distributed evenly across the large rural areas and smaller towns of Georgia. It was the conviction of most educators and mental health professionals that interdisciplinary and interagency cooperation was essential for effective and efficient use of these scattered resources. Figure 1 portrays the original array of services recognized as contributing to a comprehensive service delivery system. This figure also illustrates the range of professionals involved in cooperative planning as each local unit within the network was developed.

Local- and state-level planning was conducted by concerned individuals from these representative services. Thirteen guidelines emerged as a "platform" around which concerned agencies, advocacy

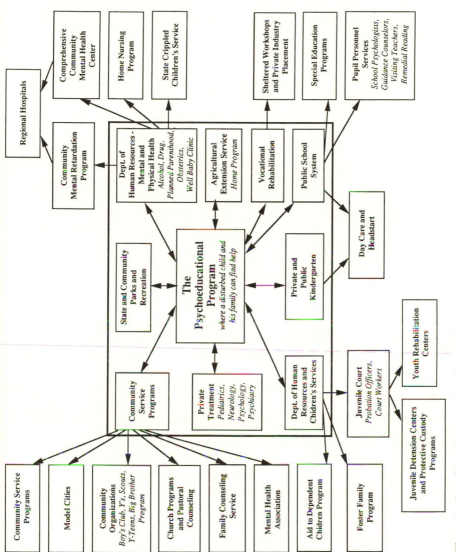

Figure 1. Coordinated services for disturbed children.

groups, legislators, and individuals built an informal coalition (Wood, 1975, p. 139). They are as follows:

1. The program should clearly distinguish mental health services for children from services for adults.
2. The program should reduce the need for hospital and residential care for young children by keeping children with their families while receiving services.
3. The program should serve children from birth to age 14 (raised to 18 years in 1979).
4. The program should keep families actively involved in supportive ways.
5. The program should keep these children, whenever possible, enrolled in a regular school or preschool program while receiving these special services.
6. The program should serve children whose problems are severe and for whom no program or service is available.
7. The program should have the qualities of both educational and mental health programs.
8. The program should draw together available professional manpower from mental health and special education.
9. The program should utilize paraprofessionals, volunteers, parents, and other community resources in the rehabilitative process.
10. The program should build upon existing agencies.
11. The program should permit counties to share services.
12. The program should be applicable to all of the rural and urban areas of the state.
13. The program should include a system for ongoing evaluation of treatment effectiveness (Wood, Quirk, & Swan, 1971).

A 13-Year Phase-In Plan

With high levels of public awareness and professionals in agreement about needed services, the network plan was designed and initiated. Thirteen years, 1969 to 1982, were required to accomplish the goal of comprehensive, statewide services to all SED children and youth and their families.

The first 3 years were used to implement a pilot program as a prototype and to replicate it in two other areas of the state (the Pilot-Demonstration phase). Three more years were needed to complete the network to 24 units serving the statewide SED population from age 2 to age 14 (Network Development phase). With the network complete, 4 additional years were used to expand program services to infants (birth to age 2) and to allow network staff to mature in their program effectiveness. Then a final 3 year expansion occurred to add services for SED youth from 15 to 18 years of age. Most current data about the completed network indicate that approximately 9,000 SED children and youth are served annually, statewide. This represents approximately one-half of 1% of the total child and youth population of the state (Jordan, 1985).

The Pilot Demonstration Phase. Funding for the original prototype, the Rutland Center, came about through the interest of a state legislator active in support of mental health programs statewide. With a written proposal for the prototype, prepared by University of Georgia faculty, educators, and local mental health professionals, he secured state funding in a special state budget line item on a year-by-year basis for the first 3 years of the demonstration project (McDaniel, Levine, & Wood, 1970). This special project, the Rutland Center, was administered by a local school district with legislative funding channeled to the local school district through the Georgia Department of Education, Division of Special Education and Pupil Personnel Services. The Georgia Department of Human Resources provided additional federal funding through the local mental health department to provide part of the clinical component. These funds were used to support services to children between the ages of 6 and 14. Additional funds were obtained by the Rutland Center director, through the University of Georgia, from the U.S. Department of Health, Education, and Welfare (HEW) Bureau for the Education of the Handicapped to provide these services to infants and preschool children (Wood, 1972c; Wood & Fendley, 1971; Wood, Quirk, & Swan, 1971).

The success of the 3-year pilot-demonstration phase was clearly documented with the program evaluation system in the original prototype. The Rutland Center program and evaluation results were given high visibility among state legislators, school leadership, mental health advocates, and parent groups. The prototype also was highlighted in the final report of the Governor's Commission to Improve Services for Mentally and Emotionally Handicapped Georgians (1971). This commission recommended statewide development of psychoeducational programs such as had been demonstrated to be effective at the Rutland Center and in replications at two other state locations. The governor responded by appointment of a staff liaison officer to serve among his office, the legislature, the involved state agencies, and the Rutland Center staff. The charge from the governor was to produce a statewide network design and a funding plan for statewide implementation. The focus on networking was designed to enhance communication, provide accountability systems, provide the equitable distribution of state resources, and assure services to all SED students and their families in Georgia.

Network Development Phase. The plan for the network was submitted to the legislature, and 14 units were approved for funding in 1972–1973. The major network objective was this:

> To serve seriously disturbed infants, children and their families by initially establishing 14 psychoeducational programs in selected regions of Georgia with outposts (miniclusters) to serve rural children geographically isolated from the proposed programs.

Figure 2 illustrates agency linkages and services to be provided. Contractual agreements between the Georgia Department of Human Resources and the Georgia Department of Education provided for the flow of designated mental health and education funds to go to local school districts that had developed proposals for operating a network unit in a designated local area. Local mental health programs were provided funds specifically in support of the clinical portion of the psychoeducational programs. Similarly, designated funds were provided by the Georgia Department of Education for the special education portion of the program.

A special line item in the state budget was established to begin the statewide network. The plan was to increase the number of units each year as state funds became available and as the designated local areas did adequate preparation and identified trained personnel to initiate such programs. The network funding also created a technical assistance office at the Rutland Center. The purpose of this office was to provide experienced consultation and staff development assistance to each local area as plans were developed for implementation of a network unit (Pettit, 1974; Wood, 1972b, 1975).

In the network design, certain essential components of the model were required for each unit, particularly, the staffing prototypes, types of services to be provided, numbers to be served, and standard program evaluation procedures to be followed. These essential components enabled the network plan to provide a fairly accurate proposal to the state legislators for annual costs and projected time lines. Areas of the state seeking to develop a unit, prepared a grant proposal following the prototype guidelines described previously, and described how the essential components would be provided. The

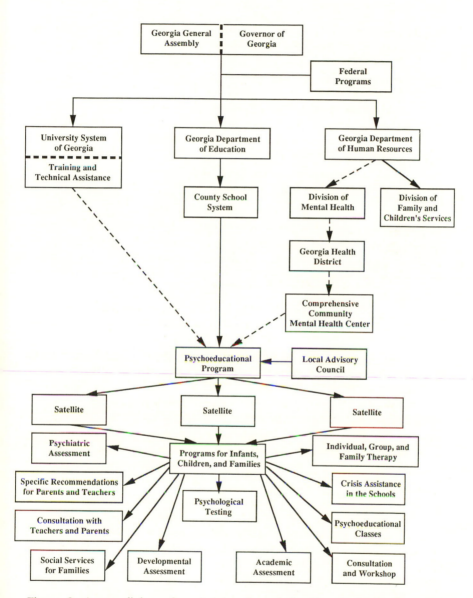

Figure 2. Agency linkage for administration of the Georgia Psychoeducational Program.

order in which the local areas of the state received funding for their units was based on satisfying four criteria:

1. There must be some existing local resources and personnel for mental health and special education.
2. There must be active interagency planning efforts within the designated geographic area.
3. Supportive resources must be available through federal funding (such as the Model Cities program providing significant assistance to poverty areas at that time).
4. The existence of high poverty rates (at least 30% of the population below the poverty level) and related conditions such as high infant mortality rates and high levels of referral to the state mental hospitals and prisons.

DESIGNING THE PROTOTYPES

Estimating the SED Prevalence

At the onset of planning for the network, census data were used to determine the number of children in each county in Georgia. From these figures, the number with severe emotional or behavioral problems was computed, using an estimate of prevalence of one-half of 1% of that population. With these figures charted on a detailed, county-by-county map of the state, a target number of potential SED children and youth in each city, town, and county was established. Although some believed this figure to be too low at the time, this method of estimating SED prevalence has proven essentially accurate for planning, funding, and service delivery over the past 15 years.

Determining the Service Areas

As planning got underway for the network, the state also was expanding its community mental health programs in response to Public Law 91-211 (1972). This law amended the Community Mental Health Centers Act to include a specific section on mental health for children (Title IV). At that time, the state was divided into 24 community mental health service delivery regions. Because these multicounty areas each had a community mental health facility and a regional psychiatric hospital with separate units for children and youth, they offered the potential for coordinated service delivery links, and therefore, the same geographic boundaries were used to delineate the areas for locating each of the psychoeducational program units to be developed for the network.

Choosing a Central Location for Each Service Area

With the state thus divided into 24 areas for psychoeducational programs, the prevalence data were examined within each area to determine the population clusters in towns and rural areas. Particular attention was given to the roads and highways, driving time, and distances between the populated areas. The result of this planning was a statewide grid showing every local school district, its roads, bus routes, child and youth population, and estimates of SED prevalence for each local school district, the multicounty areas, and throughout the state. The largest and most centrally located urban areas within each service area were tentatively designated as the central sites for each of the 24 units in the proposed network. Additional outposts, or secondary sites, were generated from each of the central sites wherever there was a child population cluster greater than 5,000.

Adjusting Unit Size to Populations

When the area boundaries were established, it was clear that certain of the 24 units would have very large SED populations, whereas other units would serve rather modest numbers. From this information, three different prototype models were designed for staffing and funding the 24 units, based on size of the total child and youth populations within each area. Table 1 outlines the numbers to be served in the three prototypes.

Type A units serve areas with a total child population of less than 30,000 (birth to age 14). Type B units serve a total child population between 30,000 and 40,000 children. Type C units serve a child population between 40,000 and 60,000. In the large metro area of the state, two Type A units and one Type B unit are used. For every outpost site operated by a central site within an area, additional personnel positions and funding are allocated to adjust for geographic differences and distances.

Staffing Prototypes by Unit Size and Service Load

The basic staffing model was designed to accomplish five interdisciplinary service functions: (a) clinical services, (b) psychoeduca-

Table 1.   How Serious Emotional Disturbances (SED) Service Loads Are Estimated According to Population and Unit Size

	Type A	Type B	Type C
	Small	Medium	Large
Child/youth population in service area	30,000 or less	31,000 to 39,000	40,000 to 60,000
SED prevalence estimate (.5% of total)	150	195	300
Services in psychoeducational classes, annually (40% of SED population)	60	78	120
Other services, annually (60% of SED population)	90	117	180
Assessment and indirect services (52% of SED population)	78	101	156
Other direct services (10% of SED population)	15	20	30

Note. The maximum population figures are used to calculate estimates.

tional therapy, (c) school and agency liaison, (d) family consultation/parent training, and (e) program evaluation. Figure 3 illustrates the general staffing prototype developed to provide these services.

The amount of staff time needed for particular service functions was established on the basis of the SED prevalence estimate for the unit. The 3 years of the pilot programs resulted in the observation that, among the accepted referrals, services in psychoeducational classes were needed for 40% of the children. The remaining 60% required other forms of more limited service, such as assistance to families, consultation with teachers, referrals and consultation with other agencies concerned with the child, and individual therapy or intermittent crisis contacts in the schools, neighborhoods, or homes. Using the 40% to 60% ratio, service load estimates were calculated. These service load estimates were then used to determine the amount of staff time needed for each service function within a unit in the network, according to size. Table 2 contains the typical staffing prototypes for each unit size. Overall network staffing also is portrayed in Table 2 with a summary of total personnel positions for 1984–1985.

To illustrate how staffing is built on service need, consider a typical Type A unit, serving an area with a child population of less than 30,000 and designed to provide referrals and assessment ser-

Administrative Personnel

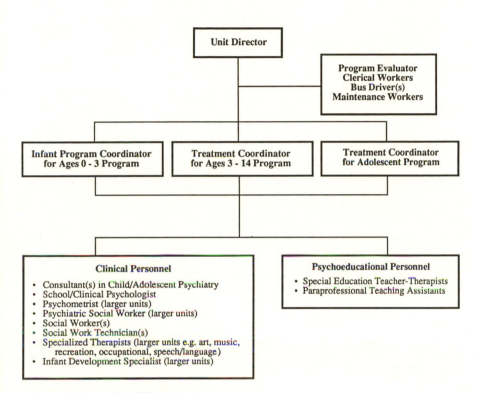

Figure 3. General staffing prototype.

vices to about 150 referred children annually (see Table 1). These referral services require staff time from the consulting psychiatrist, psychologist, social worker, educational therapist, and the treatment program coordinator (or unit director) (see Table 2). These students then require either daily psychoeducational services in classes or other intermittent service following the assessment. In a Type A unit, an estimated 60 SED children require psychoeducational classroom services (40% of the total served) and 90 SED children require some other form of service (60% of the total).

Estimating that the 60 children needing classroom service are served for an entire year, the unit would have nine special education teacher–therapists and nine paraprofessional aids to provide psychoeducational classes in groups of about seven children each. The senior

Table 2. Typical Staffing Prototypes According to Unit Size and Total Network Personnel Reported as Percentage of Full-Time Employment

	Type A Small	Type B Medium	Type C Large	Total number of network positions 1984–1985	Percentage of all personnel
Administration personnel, total				189	17
Director	100	100	100	24	
Treatment coordinators				61	
Ages 3–14 program	50	100	100		
Adolescent program	50	100	100		
Infant program	—	50	100		
Program evaluator	50	100	100	17	
Clerical	100	150	200	64	
Maintenance and bus drivers	100	150	200	23	
Clinical personnel, total				242	21
Consultant child/adolescent psychiatry	10	20	30	6	
Psychologists	30	50	200	35	
Psychometrists	—	—	100	6	
Social workers	100	200	300	82	
Social work technician(s)	—	—	—	19	
Parent workers	—	—	—	29	
Specialized therapists	—	—	—	—	
Infant development specialists	100	150	200	31	
Psychoeducational personnel, total				699	62
Special education teacher–therapists	9	11	17	349	
Paraprofessional teaching assistants	0	11	17	350	
Total network personnel				1,130	100

Note. The prototype ratio of children in classes to teacher–therapists is 7:1. In practice, this estimate fluctuates with numbers entering and exiting during a year. In 1984–1985 the annual ratio was 12 children to 1 teacher–therapist (4,318 served in classes divided by 349 teacher–therapists). Summarized from Swan (1987).

educational therapist serves as program coordinator. These teachers and aides also provide follow-up services as the children are integrated into their regular school programs.

For the 90 children and families requiring some other form of intermittent service from a Type A unit, the service load is provided by the clinical staff. About 78 of the children (52% of SED total) require assessment and forms of indirect services, whereas 15 (10%) need other forms of direct service. The senior social worker carries a case load of 60 and the half-time social work technician, a case load of 30. The psychologist, with 30% time or 12 hours per week, provides assessment, consultation to the psychoeducational program, and carries a small case load of children seen for individual therapy. The infant evaluator and social work technician specializing in infant services provide infant assessment, parent consultation, and home-based parent training programs. The consulting psychiatrist provides 4 hours a week for psychiatric evaluations to those referred children who have clinical symptoms, possible psychosis, neurological impairments, or other severe psychopathology. The psychiatrist also provides consultation to the psychoeducational program, the infant program, and to the social workers.

THE FUNDING HISTORY

Table 3 provides a summary of the funding history of the network. Data are reported in actual dollars, unadjusted for inflation. Three major resources are shown: (a) the funds contained in the state budget line item as described; (b) the number of special education teaching positions provided by the State Board of Education to be used exclusively by the local units in the network; and (c) federal funds—both P.L. 94-142, Title VI-B, and P.L. 89-313 (1966).

Table 3 shows a 150% increase in state dollars occurring during the second year of the network expansion (1973–1974), when the number of units increased by 52%. The second largest increases in funding for the network occurred during the 2-year period when the adolescent services were added (1979–1981). The most current period for which data are available (1985–1986) show a total amount of over $24 million from state and federal sources in support of this program.

The special education teaching positions reported previously in Table 2 were allocated on the basis of 40% of the SED prevalence estimates, using the staffing ratios described previously. As with state dollars, the teaching positions were increased most significantly dur-

Table 3. Network Funding History Unadjusted for Inflation

Phase	State budget dollars	Percentage annual increase	Network teaching positions from state				Funds VI-8	Funds PL89-313	Total of all sources (in dollars)
			No.	Percentage annual increase	Dollars	Percentage annual increase			
Pilot demonstration									
1969–1970	250,000	—	—	—	—	—	—	—	250,000
1970–1971	500,000	100	—	—	—	—	—	—	500,000
1971–1972	604,000	21	—	—	—	—	—	—	604,000
Network development									
1972–1973	1,071,669	77	58	—	Data not available	Data not available	—	—	1,071,669
1973–1974	2,684,000	150	88	52	Data not available	Data not available	—	—	2,684,000
1974–1975	4,292,953	60	118	34	Data not available	Data not available	—	—	4,292,953
Network completed for ages 0–14									
1975–1976	5,092,018	19	139	18	1,200,000	—	—	—	6,292,018
1976–1977	5,552,773	9	139	0	1,300,000	8	—	—	6,852,773
1977–1978	5,727,467	3	174	25	1,900,000	46	—	—	7,627,467
1978–1979	6,071,115	6	174	0	2,014,000	6	—	—	8,085,115
Network expands for ages 0–18									
1979–1980	8,228,150	36	174	0	2,200,000	9	1,391,390	185,322	12,004,862
1980–1981	11,912,323	45	174	0	2,300,000	5	2,124,065	264,431	16,600,819
1981–1982	12,829,086	8	174	0	2,610,000	13	2,182,773	425,432	18,047,291
Network completed									
1982–1983	13,552,883	6	174	0	2,784,000	—	2,213,581	436,730	18,987,194
1983–1984	13,925,126	3	174	0	3,182,000	13	2,865,317	422,951	20,345,384
1984–1985	14,665,102	5	174	0	3,306,000	6	2,865,317	437,238	21,273,647
1985–1986	17,331,545	18	174	0	3,654,000	11	2,865,305	472,335	24,323,185

aSignificant teacher/staff raise.

20

ing the final 2 years of the Network Development phase (1973–1975) when special education teaching units were increased from 58 to 118 (103%). It is interesting to note that during the second expansion of the network to provide services to adolescents in the 15–18 age group (1979–1982), additional teaching positions were not provided. The special education personnel for this expansion were supported by major allocations of P.L. 94-142, Part VI-B funds.

Not shown in Table 3 are local contributions, such as for buildings and transportation of children. Local education agencies were responsible for providing suitable housing for the central site and the outposts; however, there was no restriction on the use of grant funds to rent a facility if sufficient justification was provided. Transportation funds were provided in the state education budget to assist local school systems in the purchase of additional school busses needed to transport children to network programs.

In 1985–1986, the entire Georgia educational funding formula was changed to a student weighted formula under Georgia's Quality Basic Education Act (1985); however, the status for this network was enhanced because its funding was as a categorical grant.

STUDIES OF THE NETWORK

Recognizing the need to systematically study and utilize the vast data existing about SED children in the network, the directors of the network units, in collaboration with faculty at the University of Georgia and staff of the Georgia Department of Education, formed the Psychoeducational Program Network Research Consortium. This group conducted a series of studies to initiate an ongoing program of research, publishing the first monograph in the series in 1985, under the title, *Research Studies in the Georgia Psychoeducational Program Network* (see references by Cope, 1985; Jordan, 1985; Moffett & Moore, 1985; and Swan & Jacob, 1985). The consortium received a research grant from the U.S. Department of Education to conduct additional studies about the characteristics of the statewide SED population (Swan, 1987). The following sections of this chapter highlight some of the current findings of this Consortium effort, and describe the SED population in some detail (Swan, 1987; Swan, Purvis, & Wood, 1986; Swan, Wood, & Purvis, 1986).

Prevalence of Severe Emotional Disturbance

The original network design estimated an annual service load of one-half of 1% of the total child and youth population (the estimated rate). In 1985, the child population in the state (age 3 to 18) was 1,613,638. The network accepted 9,436 referrals for severe behavioral or emotional problems or .0058, about one-half of 1% of the child population (the actual rate). No child can be denied services because of severity of the problems alone, and there were no waiting lists for services, although time spent in the intake process, for some cases and in some locations, might be several months in duration.

Table 4 compares estimated prevalence and actual incidence rates as reflected in the network service data for 1984–1985.

Ratio of Direct to Indirect Services

The original prototype estimated that 40% of those served would require direct psychoeducational services in therapeutic classes and 60% would need other forms of service. As shown in Table 4, services in psychoeducational classes were provided in 1985 to 4,445 children, all of whom received a DSM-III diagnosis (American Psychiatric Association, 1980). This number amounted to 47% of the referrals, whereas the remaining 53% (4,991) received other services. Other services included family consultation or home-based services for parents of young children; school consultation and placement in other forms of

Table 4.   Network Service, 1984–1985 for Serious Emotional Disturbances (SED)

	Projected estimates	Actual numbers
Total child/youth population in state	—	1,613,638
SED served	8,068	9,436
Percentage of total population	.50	.58
Services in psychoeducational classes	3,227	4,445
Percentage of SED served	.40	.47
Other services, total	4,841	4,991
Percentage of SED served	.60	.53
Assessment services	4,195	5,708
Percentage of SED population	.52	.60

Note. 1980 census data, ages 3–18, statewide, adjusted for births, net in migration between 1980–1982 and out migration for those exceeding 18 years of age by 1985 (Georgia Department of Education, 1985).

special education; intermittent crisis intervention in school, home, or neighborhood; or referral and consultation with other school or agency services, particularly for children involved in the juvenile justice system or in foster homes.

Characteristics of SED Children and Youth

Children referred to a unit of the network are considered eligible when one or more of the following conditions is identified as the primary disability:

(a) Severe emotional disturbance, such as, but not limited to, schizophrenia and adjustment reactions.

(b) Severe behavioral disorders resulting from, but not limited to, autism, neurological impairment, cultural deprivation, developmental lag and family-related problems.

(c) Severe school-related problems manifested in, but not limited to, behavior, socialization, communication and academic skills. (Georgia Department of Education, 1988a, p. 88)

In a study by Swan, Purvis, and Wood (1986), of the 5,008 SED children and youth with DSM-III classifications receiving services in the network in 1984–1985, 78% were male and 22% were female. The families were about equally divided between single-parent families (41%) and families where both parents were present (46%). The remaining 13% were either in foster homes or not living with either parent.

The majority (54%) were age 9 or younger when they first received network service. There were about 200 to 300 children entering at each age between 3 years and 5 years. The number entering between 6 years and 15 years was about 300 to 400 at each age, each age representing between 6% and 7% of the total. The entrance ages for those under 5 years and over 15 were less than 6% for each age.

Diagnosis. The DSM-III provides a standard way to describe the children and youth who receive direct services in the network. Principal diagnosis according to DSM-III is "the condition that was chiefly responsible for occasioning the evaluation or admission" (American Psychiatric Association, 1980, p. 24). For summary purposes, DSM-III diagnoses of the 5,008 SED children and youth in the sample were grouped into 12 broad categories and are reported in Table 5.

The largest group of children were diagnosed for evaluation or admission as having adjustment disorders (24%). This included children with excessive maladaptive reactions to identified psychosocial stressors resulting in impairment in social functioning, for example,

**Table 5. Summary of DSM-III
Primary Diagnoses for Evaluation or
Admission of 5,008 Serious Emotional
Disturbances (SED) in Children and
Youth in 1984–1985**

Category	Number	Percentage of total
Adjustment dis- orders	1,190	24
Conduct disor- ders	959	19
Attention defi- cit disorders	685	14
Autism	357	7
Personality dis- orders	312	6
Anxiety/ avoidance disorders	310	6
Developmental learning problems	262	5
Affective/mood disorders	252	5
Mental retarda- tion	232	5
Psychoses	203	4
Organic mental disorders and substance abuse	48	1
Diagnois in- complete	198	4
Total	5,008	100

Note. From Swan (1987).

adjustment disorders, 309.xx; elective mutism, 313.23; oppositional disorders, 313.81; reactive attachment disorders, 313.89; parent–child problems, v61.20; other specified family circumstances, v61.80; and phase of life problems, v62.89.

The second most frequently occurring diagnosis for evaluation or admission was in the conduct disorders category (*n* = 959 or 19%), including problems of repetitive and persistent patterns of behavior in which the rights of other or major age-appropriate societal norms are violated, not caused by personality disorder. Included in this group were conduct disorders and impulse control problems (coded 312.XX). The Georgia definition of SED specifically excludes students who, as a single presenting diagnosis, are socially maladjusted. This is consistent with federal definitions.

The third most frequently occurring diagnosis for evaluation or admission was in the attention deficit disorders category (n = 685 or 14%). This group included developmentally inappropriate attention seeking, excessive motor activity, and impulsivity (coded 314.XX).

Services. About one-half of the 5,008 SED children and youth in the sample received network services at main locations (52%), with the remainder served at rural outpost locations (48%). Preschool programs were provided to 11%; elementary programs to 58% (age range 5–14); and programs for adolescents comprised 31% (ages 15 to 19). Most of the direct services for this sample were through therapeutic psychoeducational classes (80%). Other forms of individual counseling or therapy to child or parent were provided to 17%, and direct assistance in regular schools was provided to 3%.

The median length of time the children received network services was 17 months; however, there was considerable variation, reflected in an average of 24 months (11% received services for 4 years or more).

Exit Data. During 1984–1985, 1,928 (38% of the sample) exited from network programs. Almost two-thirds (61%) of these had made sufficient progress as to no longer need network services or to warrant exit to other, less intensive services. The remaining 39% of the exits were caused by circumstances such as family moves or placement of adolescents in juvenile correction programs.

In this sample, those exiting the network went to a wide range of placements. About 20% (387) returned directly to regular education programs and did not require further special assistance. Less than 6% were placed in more restrictive settings such as youth development centers, regional mental hospitals, or private residential schools, whereas 38% returned to special education classes in the public schools; 35% were withdrawn or dropped out, and subsequent placements were unknown.

In another study of 382 children exiting the network because they had been judged to have achieved program objectives and no longer in need of network services, Swan and Jacob (1985) found that 34% of the placements at exit were into regular education classes. Thirty-one percent of the children went to special education resource rooms and self-contained special education classes. Approximately 28% were placed in special education self-contained classes. Approximately the same number exited in 1 year from the network's preschool, primary, elementary, and middle-school-age groups, whereas exits among adolescents were greater. This latter finding may reflect decreasing enrollments in adolescent programs due to voluntary dropouts at age 18.

Recidivism

Recidivism among the group studied by Swan and Jacob (1985) was 13% (639 children during 1985–1986 who had previously exited and then returned for services). Approximately one-half of those who had exited previously did so for circumstantial reasons, either moving elsewhere or being withdrawn by parents without the recommendation of network staff.

Longitudinal Effect

A follow-up study of 64 students 3 to 5 years after exiting network programs indicated that 51% did not need any special education services in 3 to 5 years following their exit (Moffett & Moore, 1985). Specifically, 47% ($n = 30$) were in one of the following: (a) regular education placements ($n = 15$), (b) postsecondary placements ($n = 2$), or (c) working ($n = 13$). In this follow-up group, 25 were adolescents, 13 or 52% of whom were successfully employed.

Academic Achievement and IQ

To study typical IQ levels and academic achievements, 344 children were selected for a stratified random sample of the total group receiving direct network services in 1984–1985 (Swan, 1987). The sample was selected to represent the proportion of children in the preschool, elementary, and adolescent programs. The sample also represented proportional distributions of sex and DSM-III categories. The average school-grade placement for the total network population was third grade, and the average age was 9 years. These same proportions also were reflected in the selected sample. Academic achievement scores showed them to be at grade level or better; that is, achieving at or above the expected third grade level. For example, 203 students were tested on the PIAT and achieved an average reading score for grade 4.6 ($SD = 4.7$) and an average math score for grade 4.4 ($SD = 2.8$). Somewhat similar scores were achieved by 55 students in the sample using the Brigance and achieving an average reading score of grade 4.6 ($SD = 2.9$).

Using the WISC-R, a mean IQ score of 81 ($SD = 18$) was obtained for 220 students in the sample. On the Stanford–Binet, the mean IQ was 66 ($SD = 22$) for 44 students; and on the Kaufman, 4 students earned an average IQ score of 100 ($SD = 13$). This contrast between grade-appropriate achievement and lowered IQ scores suggests that measurement of these variables may be confounded by severe emotional disturbance.

A similar result was obtained by Cope (1985) in a study of the academic progress of 137 SED students in the network. His results indicate that SED students made from 6½ to 8½ months of academic progress during a school year while enrolled in a network program, with a range of 2 months to 18 months, depending on the instrument used to measure achievement.

Personnel

The quality of personnel is a vital component for effective psychoeducational service delivery. At a minimum, program staff should possess an appropriate educational background and the ability to meet certification requirements for their positions. Experience also is an important consideration. The Network Research Consortium conducted a study in 1986 (Swan, Wood, & Purvis, 1986) on the staffing quality among the 1,130 network personnel (see Table 2). The positions in the network were grouped into three categories, according to major service function:

1. Psychoeducational classroom personnel, such as special education teacher–therapists and aides, who provide direct service on a sustained basis.
2. Clinical personnel, such as psychiatrists, psychologists, infant program workers, social workers, and a number of specialty therapists (occupational, speech/language, art, music, recreation, etc.), who provide therapeutic services on an intermittent basis as supplements to the daily psychoeducational services.
3. Administrative personnel who provide backup assistance and leadership but do not personally provide services, including unit directors, program coordinators, secretaries, program evaluators, maintenance workers, and bus drivers.

A summary of the findings of the Swan, Wood, and Purvis (1986) study concerning the education, credentials, and experience of the network personnel is provided in the following section.

Psychoeducational Classroom Personnel. Of the 315 teacher–therapists in the network, all had been graduated with a college degree and 142 (45%) had earned a Master's degree. Their certification levels generally followed their academic degree levels and 271 (86%) had certification specifically in the education of emotionally disturbed or behavior disordered students. Another 8% had certification in other areas of special education, whereas the remaining 5% held certificates in various areas of general education. As a group, they had an average of 5 years experience in the field and 4½ years of work in the network.

Clinical Personnel. There were 234 clinical personnel in the network in 1984–1985. Of these, 218 (93%) had 4-year college degrees and 104 (44%) held a Master's degree. A doctoral degree was held by 16 (7%) of the clinical personnel. Ninety-six percent held certification in their specialization fields. The clinical personnel generally had more years of work experience than the psychoeducational classroom personnel, with an average of 6 years work with SED children and youth. Most of this experience had come from their work in the network.

Administrative Personnel. Among the 24 unit directors, all held Master's degrees or higher. Post-Master's degrees were held by 79%. Their areas of certification included administration (38%), psychology (25%), special education for SED children (25%), school psychology (8%), and counseling (4%).

There were 56 treatment coordinators in the network. Typically, the larger units in the network had separate coordinators for preschool, elementary, and adolescent programs, whereas smaller units had only one or two program coordinators. All but one coordinator had a Master's degree or higher. Their area of certification reflected their academic degrees with 64% in the area of special education for SED children, 11% in psychology, 7% in other special education areas, 7% in counseling, 5% in social work, 4% in early childhood, and 2% in psychometry.

Among all network personnel, those in administrative positions had the longest employment record in the network, with an average of 7.3 years. This finding may be related to the "burnout" factor less often affecting administrative personnel than direct service personnel, who work on a daily basis for sustained time periods with SED children.

SUMMARY AND CONCLUSION

The Georgia Psychoeducational Network has demonstrated its viability and effectiveness as a statewide program of mental health and special education services for severely emotionally disturbed and seriously behaviorally disordered children and youth and their families. Its structure and long-term development, based on the combination of public and professional concerns and implemented by combined support from both mental health and education at the local, state, and university levels, provide a model for others to consider as they develop effective and viable services for these children and youth and their families.

The collaboration among local agencies, state agencies, and the university system combined with the priority on accountability and program evaluation are an effective vehicle for the network to continue to examine its efforts and determine the most effective ways to serve these children and youth and their families based on the latest findings. The emphasis on local flexibility within statewide parameters provides a proven effective means for the statewide program to continue to refine its efforts to provide the highest quality services within the context of local resources.

REFERENCES

American Psychiatric Association. (1980). *Diagnostic and statistical manual of mental disorders* (3rd ed.). Washington, DC: Author.

Apter, S. J. (1982). *Troubled children: Troubled systems.* New York: Pergamon Press.

Blom, S. D., Lininger, R. S., & Charlesworth, W. R. (1987). Ecological observation of emotionally and behaviorally disordered students: An alternative method. *American Journal of Orthopsychiatry, 57,* 49–59.

Cope, T. H. (1985). Academic progress of SED students served in the Georgia Psychoeducational Program Network. *Research studies in the Georgia Psychoeducational Program Network.* Research Report #85-101:5–9.

Georgia Department of Education (1985). *Georgia Psychoeducational Network Annual Report.* Atlanta: Program for Exceptional Children.

Georgia Department of Education (1988a). *Regulations and procedures.* Atlanta: Program for Exceptional Children.

Georgia Department of Education (1988b). *Psychoeducational Directors Handbook.* Atlanta: Program for Exceptional Children.

Georgia's Quality Basic Education Act. (1985). Atlanta: Georgia Department of Education, Office of Superintendent.

Gottlieb, B. H. (1981). (Ed.). *Social network and social support.* Beverly Hills: Sage Publishers.

Governor's Commission to Improve Services for Mentally and Emotionally Handicapped Georgians. (1971). The Honorable John L. Moore, Jr., Chairman, *Final Report by the Commission.* Atlanta: Georgia Archives, June 23, 1971, Author.

Hunter, A., & Riger, S. (1986). The meaning of community in community mental health. *Journal of Community Psychology, 14,* 55–71.

Jordan, J. A. (1985). Introduction and overview. *Research studies in the Georgia Psychoeducational Program Network.* (Report No. 101:1–4).

McDaniel, C., Levine, L., & Wood, M. M. (1970). *A psychoeducational center for emotionally disturbed children: A community model.* Working paper. Unpublished manuscript.

Moffett, N. W., & Moore, G. (1985). Longitudinal followup of students three to five years after termination from programs in the Georgia Psychoeducational Program Network. *Research studies in the Georgia Psychoeducational Program Network.* Research Report #85-101:17–22.

Pettit, P. (1974). The Georgia Psychoeducational Network. In *Total mental health services in Georgia* (pp. 19–26). Atlanta: Metropolitan Cooperative Educational Service Agency.

Platt, J. (1973). The Rutland Center. In *Exemplary programs for the handicapped: Vol. 3. Early childhood education case studies* (AAI Report No. 73–84). Cambridge, MA: Abstract Associates.

Public Law 89-313, Amendments to Elementary and Secondary Education Act, 1966.

Public Law 91-211, Amendments to Community Mental Health centers Act, 1972.

Public Law 94-142, Education for All Handicapped Children Act of 1975, November 29, 1975.

Public Law 98-199, Education of the Handicapped Amendments of 1983, December 2, 1983.

Public Law 99-457, Education of the Handicapped Amendments of 1986, October 8, 1986.

Swan, W. W. (1987). Final Report—*The Georgia Psychoeducational Program Network Research Consortium.* Research Project, Field Initiated studies, Research Projects Branch, Office of Special Education Services, U.S. Department of Education, Grant #G008530255.

Swan, W. W., & Jacob, R. T. (1985). Provisionally terminated students in Georgia: Where are they? *Research Studies in the Georgia Psychoeducational Program Network.* Research Report #85-101:10–16.

Swan, W. W., Purvis, J. W., & Wood, N. J. (1986). *A quantitative study of Georgia SED students: A working paper.* Athens: The University of Georgia, Unpublished manuscript.

Swan, W. W., Wood, N. J., & Purvis, J. W. (1986). *Personnel in the Georgia Psychoeducational Network: A working paper.* Athens: The University of Georgia. Unpublished manuscript.

Walker, H. M. (1982). Assessment of behavior disorders in the school setting: Issues, problems, and strategies. In M. M. Noel & N. G. Haring (Eds.), *Progress or change: Issues in educating the emotionally disturbed: Vol. 1: Identification and program planning* (pp. 11–42). Seattle: Program Development Assistance Systems.

Wood, M. M. (1972a). *The Rutland Center model for treating emotionally disturbed children.* Athens: Rutland Center Technical Assistance Office.

Wood, M. M. (1972b). An example of program development and the replication process. In D. W. Davis, B. Elliott, & R. R. DeVoid (Eds.), *Replication guidelines* (pp. 28–36). Chapel Hill: Technical Assistance Development System, The University of North Carolina.

Wood, M. M. (1972c). *Rutland Center: Psychoeducational Center for the Northeast Georgia Health District: Funding proposal.* Unpublished manuscript.

Wood, M. M. (1975). A case study in replication: Replicating services for young handicapped children. In L. Gunn & D. Davis (Eds.), *Outreach* (pp. 133–153). Chapel Hill, NC: Technical Assistance Development Systems, The University of North Carolina.

Wood, M. M., & Fendley, A. L. (1971). A community psychoeducational center for emotionally disturbed children. *Focus on Exceptional Children, 3,* 9–11.

Wood, M. M., Quirk, J. P., & Swan, W. W. (1971). *Current services to children with serious emotional and behavioral problems in Georgia: A current status summary report: A report to the Governor's Commission to Improve Services for Mentally and Emotionally Handicapped Georgians,* The Honorable John L. Moore, Jr., Chairman. Georgia Archives, June 23, 1971.

Zabel, R. H., Peterson, R. L., Smith, C. R., & White, M. A. (1982). Availability and usefulness of assessment information for emotionally disabled students. *School Psychology Review, 11,* 433–437.

2

Start-Up of a Day Treatment Program in a University Medical Center

LAUREL J. KISER and DAVID B. PRUITT

INTRODUCTION

University medical centers have the complex and expensive responsibility to provide medical education. In order to meet this mandate, they must attract quality medical academicians and students through the initiation and operation of excellent clinical programs. In addition to this responsibility for education, they are also committed to research endeavors and are becoming more dependent on programs that have the potential to support clinical faculty and to operate with fiscal independence. Child and adolescent day treatment programs provide an innovative clinical approach able to support educational opportunities, research programs, and clinical services. The mesh among university objectives and day treatment potentials allows medical universities to provide one of a variety of settings in which the operation of a child and adolescent day treatment program is appropriate.

Here we will provide some insight and information on starting a day treatment program for children and adolescents within a university medical center. This is not intended as a "how-to" manual because each program is unique and will require individual structuring in

LAUREL J. KISER and DAVID B. PRUITT • Day Treatment Program, University of Tennessee, Memphis, Tennessee 38105.

order to fit within the existing system. This discussion is intended to provide the benefits of experience: ideas and suggestions about what is negative, what is possible, and what is impossible in a successful university child and adolescent day treatment program.

This chapter contains a brief history of our start-up, a discussion of the relationship of the university's goals to the program (clinical, teaching, research, and fiscal), and sections dealing with using the system, with facilities management and with the university's bureaucracy. Each section covers the unique aspects of operating a child and adolescent day treatment program within a medical setting.

BRIEF HISTORY OF OUR EXPERIENCE

In September 1982, several members of the Division of Child and Adolescent Psychiatry, Department of Psychiatry, University of Tennessee Center for Health Sciences became interested in the concept of day treatment. Space for such a program was available in the building housing the division. No comparable service was available in the community, and the department chairperson, the chancellor, and the dean were willing to consider sponsoring a new program. The university's interest in starting a day treatment program was multifaceted and included (a) developing a model program, (b) creating a population that could serve as the a base for teaching and research, (c) utilizing available space, and (d) capitalizing on the potential for financial solvency.

Funding state-supported institutions in 1982 was a losing battle; even heavily supported programs saw an erosion of their funding bases. Consequently, the university was supporting the initiation of new programs only under very limited conditions. Therefore, the original contract negotiated between the Division of Child Psychiatry and the university contained the following provisions:

> The university would pay for all renovations to the space ($16,000); the university would fund the program director's position for a period of 1 year ($27,000); the university would provide an interest-free loan for start-up costs ($40,000); the Day Treatment Program would generate sufficient funds to repay the loan and be self-supporting after the first year.

RELATIONSHIP OF THE UNIVERSITY'S GOALS
TO THE DAY TREATMENT PROGRAM

As in any large organization, successful programs and the responsibilities of faculty and staff are determined by the major goals of the university. In any medical university, three of these goals are always clinical service, teaching, and the scholarly activities of research, writing, and publication. A program that supports all of these goals has an excellent opportunity for success in a university setting. A day treatment program is just such a program.

The emphasis of the day treatment program will depend to a certain extent on the program's mission as defined by the university. If the university is interested in sponsoring a teaching and research program, these areas will have top priority. If the university sets a goal of economic self-sufficiency, clinical services will be the focal point of program policy decisions. The main goals of the university are reflected in faculty responsibilities of the day treatment program team members. In addition to clinical responsibilities for day treatment patients, faculty are expected to be actively involved in teaching and research activities.

Clinical Aspects

A university medical center must provide excellent opportunities in both academic and clinical experiences for its faculty and students. A day treatment program for children and adolescents presents the opportunity for a division of child psychiatry to operate a strong clinical program. However, the clinical aspects of a day treatment program within a university medical center must be consistent with the philosophy of both the department and the clinical faculty.

The maxim "When in Rome . . ." applies to operating a clinical program within a medical center. Use of a medical model in the clinical management of day treatment patients helps the program to more closely meet the capabilities and needs of the students, faculty, and staff. This requires the active involvement of medical personnel, namely child psychiatrists, through the use of the biopsychosocial model of treatment. (For further information on this model, see the chapter by the authors, A Systems Model of Day Treatment.)

The clinical management of a program within a university medical center will differ according to each university's objective for the program. Obviously, effective clinical management is a goal for any successful program. However, the extent to which other decisions will revolve around clinical issues depends upon the goals of the medical university as a whole. In our setting, fiscal solvency was a major goal of the program. For this reason, patient care and customer satisfaction became the first objectives of the program. Other aspects, that is, teaching and research, were essential but secondary to clinical considerations.

Teaching Aspects

Affiliation with a university carries the responsibility of providing educational experiences above and beyond clinical services. Use of the multidisciplinary team approach provides a built-in opportunity for learning. Each team member is exposed to the ideas of other staff members and has access to the experience and knowledge of senior faculty.

A day treatment rotation also provides a built-in opportunity for education. The rotation is geared to the individual trainee's needs and includes experiences ranging from observing the milieu setting to co-therapy with group or families and providing therapies directly. Moreover, each student, regardless of the level of her or his training, is supervised individually by a staff/faculty member in the trainee's discipline.

Medical students, adult psychiatry residents, child psychiatry fellows, psychology interns, nursing students, social work interns, graduate students in special education and recreational therapy, and others have clinical training needs that can be met through a day treatment rotation. In fact, the day treatment setting provides a unique training opportunity in that it introduces students to an alternative to outpatient and inpatient treatment.

In addition, a day treatment program can offer summer intern positions for undergraduate students with interests in children, education, psychiatry, and psychology. These students can be paid to function as psychiatric technicians and assist the direct care staff in structuring activities for the patients. They also have the opportunity to attend several weekly conferences and seminars with other trainees and can have various other standard training experiences. These positions can serve as an important employee/trainee function.

A formal emphasis on educational opportunities for the staff can also be provided. Staff and faculty can be encouraged to participate in continuing educational experiences. Involvement in ongoing conferences, lectureships, courses, and grand rounds offered by the department or the university can be supported. When necessary, this encouragement can be backed by funding built into the program budget. Other examples of educational opportunities include staff development activities directed toward the entire staff and faculty involved in the program. Finally, some tuition discounts or subsidies can be offered staff and faculty who wish to take job-related course work. These functions, although possible in a nonuniversity setting, should be much more accepted and encouraged in a university program.

Advantages

Operating as a training facility can have advantages and disadvantages for the treatment program as well as for the trainees. The most important advantage is the exposure of future professionals to a severely neglected and underutilized treatment modality. Most mental health professionals complete their training without knowledge of or experience in alternatives to outpatient or inpatient treatment. A day treatment rotation enables the trainee to learn which patients can benefit from day treatment and the advantages and limitations of therapy in a day treatment setting. This, in turn, lends support to the day treatment system, indirectly benefiting all participants in that system.

Other advantages are more tangible; they benefit the program as it functions every day. An example is the increase in staff to patient ratio. A trainee's experience must include some clinical services; therefore he or she may provide some additional staff coverage during on-unit activities and off-unit trips or may provide additional therapy to individuals, groups, and families.

An increase in morale and motivation is another potential advantage. Trainees frequently have new ideas and approaches for dealing with patients or improving the program milieu. Often these new ideas can be successfully incorporated into the program. This sense of growth can spread to the permanent staff, increasing their commitment and decreasing their feelings of burnout. Finally, there are increased opportunities for the staff and faculty of the day treatment program to be involved in supervision.

Disadvantages

A realistic overview of training responsibilities also includes disadvantages for a day treatment program. The considerable staff time required for coordinating, supervising, and monitoring the rotation is one such drawback. It can be argued that the additional clinical services provided by inexperienced trainees does not compensate for the time required of the more experienced staff. The use of inexperienced staff may drive some patients (families) away from treatment.

Student impermanence also causes some difficulties for the program. The treatment team is forced to go through many transitions, welcoming, adjusting to, and bidding farewell to many trainees in a relatively short time. This can cause some problems. Additionally, if students pick up cases to follow in therapy, transition problems can arise. Patients must then adjust to a new therapist. If the trainee's rotation is shorter than the patient's stay in the program, the patient might have to make this adjustment more than once. For this reason, advanced trainees involved in therapy can be limited to rotations of 4 months or longer.

Research Aspects

In a university, all tenures, promotions, and raises are based to some extent (usually a great extent) on scholarly writings and publications. A day treatment program is a rich mine for such activities for several reasons. It provides a treatment model to evaluate and compare, a stable, accessible patient population to study, and an economic concept to examine. It also provides a wealth of research topics; there are few published data on treatment effectiveness, program evaluations, treatment comparisons, and cost efficiency.

This research benefits the day treatment program as well as the university by creating a good mesh for the university's needs and goals and those of the program. This leads to greater university support of the program, which, in turn, enhances the resources that can be spent studying the day treatment model. Additionally, it can stimulate growth and change within the program. Clinical benefits from a research and program evaluation emphasis include continuous monitoring of program and treatment effectiveness, quality assurance, utilization review, and peer review. Problems that are raised, analyzed, and discussed may lead to program modifications and improvements.

Another benefit is the clinical application of research data in treatment by using accepted instruments for measuring psychopathology and change. Diagnostic information, intrapsychic dynamics, and family constellations may show up on research instruments and can be applied clinically to the individual child/adolescent family to enhance treatment. Note: With this approach, care must be taken in designing the research so that the use of information from research records in treatment does not jeopardize the integrity of the research results.

Finally, staff involvement and acknowledgment in assessment, analysis, and publication can provide an increased awareness of therapeutic issues, treatment effectiveness, and program success. Moreover, it can help motivate the staff to maintain quality treatment and obtain accurate data.

In designing research protocols to be used in a clinical setting, it is necessary to balance the clinical involvement of the staff and faculty responsible for additional research activities and to balance the importance of research against the importance of treatment. Decisions must be made and priorities established. These decisions determine what data is to be collected, who will be involved in data collection, and how the results of research instruments will be used.

Fiscal Aspects

University medical centers provide some unique opportunities to generate fiscal support for a child and adolescent day treatment program. Sharing of manpower, space, and the like provides ways of subsidizing the program. For instance, the child psychiatrist with clinical responsibilities for day treatment might be paid from university funds rather than from program funds. This can be extended to a variety of faculty and staff members, especially those who carry joint responsibilities. We mention shared use of facilities here because it affects the fiscal operation of the program. However, it is discussed extensively in the next section. Table 1 presents several yearly budgets indicating (among other things) the amount of revenue contributed by the university.

Establishing the program within a medical program allows for billing on a "fee-for-service" basis. This means a higher dependence on medical insurance for reimbursement of program costs. Again referring to Table 1, note that the majority of our revenue is from third party payments.

USING THE SYSTEM

There are numerous options for ownership of a day treatment program for children and adolescents within a university medical setting. Two of the most obvious are within a department of psychiatry: the Division of Child and Adolescent Psychiatry and the Division of Psychology. Placement within either division will meet some departmental goals, that is operating a clinical service, supporting faculty and staff salaries with monies generated within the department, and placing trainees.

Wherever the program is located, liaison with other specialties is a must and a major benefit of operating within a university system. Nursing, pediatrics, developmental disabilities, speech and hearing education, and social work can provide important support services to the day treatment staff. Collaboration with any of these disciplines

**Table 1.   Start-Up Budget, 1982–1983, and
Sample Budget, 1985–1986**

	Start-up budget	1985–1986 budget
Expenses		
Personnel salaries	$76,166	$187,152
Staff benefits	19,042	46,464
Total payroll	$95,208	$233,616
Travel	1,000	1,500
Printing		700
Communications	1,500	1,200
Repairs	1,000	250
Food	11,040	
Professional services	1,000	15,000
Supplies	13,150	8,000
Rentals	24,000	23,000
Contractual		10,800
Other expenditures	2,000	1,000
Total operating expense	$54,690	$62,050
Equipment and furniture	12,120	5,000
Total expenses	$162,018	$300,666
Revenue		
Dean's office	$40,000	
Director's salary	33,750	
Medicaid, private pay, insurance	88,268	$269,051
Donated university MEM	——	31,615
	$162,018	$300,666

Note. MEM = materials, equipment, maintenance.

might include consultations on difficult patients, referrals both to and from the program, joint research projects, and placement of trainees.

For example, in our program, we tried several ways of providing the nursing care our patients required. We hired a full-time psychiatric nurse; we utilized physicians in this capacity and we managed without nursing care for short periods of time. Finally we developed a consulting relationship with a group of nurses already employed by the university in another program. They are able to provide nursing intakes, daily medication rounds, and emergency consultation as needed.

FACILITIES MANAGEMENT

Space is a significant concern in a university. Buildings are extremely expensive to construct, and available land is scarce on many university campuses. Consequently, the use of space becomes a major issue involving status as well as economics. Quantity of space must be matched by quality and usability.

Obtaining appropriate space is a first priority in any start-up negotiations. Because space is at such a premium in most universities, there usually is a considerable amount of red tape and committee structure to overcome to reach even a slight understanding of what space is available. With this recognition, one must be creative in getting access to this space. One possible strategy is to offer improvements and maintenance in exchange for access. Another is to pay rent at a reasonable, yet below-market-value rate.

Gaining access to university space is worth the effort involved because a university offers many space and facility advantages to a day treatment program. Often there are opportunities to use exceptional space and physical facilities at little or no cost to the program. For example, therapy rooms, such as video rooms, group rooms, play rooms, and the like might be shared by existing outpatient and inpatient programs and the new day treatment program. Coordination of scheduling and responsibility for maintenance of such areas are relatively simple to arrange.

Recreational space, an important consideration in a child and adolescent program, is usually difficult to obtain and costly. Many times there are existing university programs with outside play/recreational areas. Shared use of these facilities can often be arranged. For instance, the patients in the latency-age group of our day treatment program enjoy spending some activity periods on the playground of the university's Child Development Center. Student athletic facilities are another potential resource for recreational space. Use of the gym, swimming pool, racquet ball courts, and equipment expands the scope of physical activities available to day treatment patients. In some universities, rental fees for the use of athletic facilities may have to be incorporated into the program's budget. Negotiation of such fees can often lead to rates considerably lower than those required by commercial facilities. Other creative ideas include using student center facilities. Student cafeterias or university food services are sometimes willing to accommodate patients and staff as part of their catering services either on a regular basis or as occasional guests in the cafeteria. For our patients, for example, eating lunch in the student center cafeteria twice a week is one of their earned privileges.

THE UNIVERSITY BUREAUCRACY

The strength of any good program is its ability to maximize the advantages and minimize the disadvantages inherent in its setting. Dealing with the university bureaucracy presents just such a challenge.

There are many components of a university that can expedite the establishment of a new program. These include such things as human resources, legal services, secretarial and support staff, and maintenance. The development office should also be included in this list. The personnel therein can provide a variety of services including public relations, publicity, a network with community resources, and information about the university's strategies and procedures for raising funds. They should also provide guidance to the new program to ensure a coordinated effort by the university in interacting with the community. This protects community support for the university as a whole and extends it to the day treatment program specifically.

In addition to these advantages, working with a university bureaucracy requires finesse, patience, and tolerance of human error. But, as previously indicated, it is worth the extra effort in order to have a day treatment program in a medical university setting.

CONCLUSION

Day treatment programs for children and adolescents have a difficult history characterized largely by underutilization and struggles for survival. It seems important for such programs to have strong backing and support in order to succeed. A university medical center is able to provide such support. Support in this context does not mean financial assistance; a good program is able to support itself financially. A university provides support in numerous other ways that are more valuable to the survival of the program. The wise day treatment administrator will begin his or her program with cautious knowledge of the strengths and weaknesses of the university support system.

3

Architectural Considerations in Planning a Day Treatment Center

VICTOR HORNBEIN

THE ROLE OF ARCHITECTURE

The Fundamental Function

The fundamental task of architecture is to place itself between people and the natural environment in which they find themselves, in such a way as to modify the effects of environmental factors that act directly on the human body. Because of the continuous fluctuation of all environmental factors across time, the building shell must be visualized not as a simple barrier but rather as a selective, permeable membrane with the capability to admit, reject, or filter any of these factors. The roof must shed rain, withstand heavy snow loads, provide shade. The walls must resist wind, rain, cold, heat, and still admit light and air.

This fundamental requirement, however, must be integrated with the visual attributes of the nonverbal art of architecture, the attributes that elicit particular feelings or aesthetic responses. It is not possible to describe verbally how the elements can be assembled to educe a particular response. The task, a gratifying one, must be left to the architect to conceive and reduce to graphic delineation, the means

VICTOR HORNBEIN • 266 Jackson Street, Denver, Colorado 80206.

to the desired end—the reality of the building. Far from being narrowly based upon any single sense of perception such as vision, our response to a building derives from the body's total response to its perception of the environmental and functional conditions that that building affords. Function, in its broadest sense, aesthetics, and structure form an integrated whole. The functional arrangement is a correlative determinant of both structure and aesthetics, each within its modifiable limits, determining the others. The three-dimensional spatial qualities evoking the emotional responses required by the programmed use and the most efficient structural system grow from the architect's plan. The three-way relationship is analogous to the living form: It is analogically organic. The plan is the solution; the three dimensional reality is the expression.

The Aesthetic Constituent

As the functional element includes the environmentally optimal conditions, the aesthetic includes the properties of form, spatial quality, scale, proportion, balance, rhythm, texture, and color. The creative process interweaves and integrates, and all is inextricably an essential part of the whole—the reality of the building.

Form. Architectural form, the three-dimensional conformation of the building, derives from external environmental forces acting upon it, the organization of functional spaces within it, the rational structural system that supports it, the materials of which it is built, and the expression of its function, all acting as correlative determinants. The creative process of design begins with the plan, which involves the orderly arrangement of the various functional spaces most suitable to the proposed use of the building and the comfort and pleasure of the users. Additionally, the functional spaces must be so arranged that both externally and internally there is a perception of balance, symmetric or asymmetric, and its correlate, proportion.

Balance and proportion, as necessary attributes of form, are visual perceptions that can elicit feelings of comfort, stability, shelter, quiescence or, conversely, activity, energy, motion, and even frenzy. Careful attention must be directed to the proportioning and balancing of forms and elements so as to evoke the desired emotional response.

Simplicity, emphasized in most discussions of architectural aesthetics, has created a serious misconception, the consequence of which is the many prosaic lifeless buildings seen everywhere. Simplicity in architecture is indeed a virtue, but it is the simplicity of the organic—the seemingly simple form of a leaf, or a flower, or the body of an animal, which, at closer sight, is found to be composed of very many functioning parts, subtly articulated, but always integral parts of the whole. Aesthetic simplicity, a satisfaction to the mind when valid and profound, derives from inner complexity—the complexity of the several related and diverse functions that are implicitly or explicitly expressed three dimensionally.

Spatial Quality. Space is the essence of architecture, aesthetic as well as utilitarian, external as well as internal. It is defined, limited, and given subjective meaning by the enclosing or partially enclosing vertical, horizontal, or slanting planes of walls, floors, and ceilings internally and by adjacent buildings or landscape elements externally. Space is characterized not only by the three dimensions of length, breadth, and height but by the fourth dimension of time as well. As one moves around, about, and through a building, in however short a period of time, the relation of elements changes, one to the other. New visual arrangements and compositions appear and change again as other elements come into view; the rhythm of replicated parts forms new rhythms; the space becomes vibrant and alive.

When function requires relatively small spaces, the spatial quality must be imparted to each small space by treatment of enclosing planes such that each space is felt to be a part of the whole rather than an isolated, unrelated box or cell. If upper parts of partitions are glazed, ceilings will have continuity thereby visually relating spaces, and the small rooms requiring aural and visual privacy will lose the feeling of constriction that they otherwise would have. The interplay of the vertical planes of walls and partitions with the horizontal or slanting planes of ceilings of various heights also will enhance the spatial quality.

Scale. The scale of a building—the perceived relation in size to the human figure—is of immense importance, particularly of a building designed for the use of children. Space is given scale by the enclosing planes designed with three-dimensional qualities, sized to conform or harmonize with the human body in such a way as to allow the users to feel themselves in consonance with the building and to participate comfortably in its spaces and forms. The treatment center should be scaled to the children and harmonize with the appropriately dimensioned furniture and fixtures for the age group. The difference in scale from the conventional must be subtle, for the adults, too, must feel comfortable. Required is a sensitive eye and a skilled hand to achieve the desired result.

Materials. The materials used, both externally and internally, play a significant role in creating the desired perceptions of the building's purpose and will, themselves, effect an emotional response. Masonry walls, interior as well as exterior, convey a feeling of strength, permanence, and security. Fieldstone or uncoursed ledgerock, available in a variety of earth colors, relates well to a rural or suburban location but feels inappropriate in built-up urban areas. Coursed cut stone is suitable in an urban setting but is, perhaps, too formal and stately for a children's center. Brick masonry has good scale for the purpose, can be had in a wide range of earth colors and textures, is compatible with most settings, and is aesthetically pleasing when used for interior walls and partitions.

Wood siding, clapboards, or shingles, stained rather than painted, are warm and friendly and feel lighter, less ponderous than masonry, and can be had with noncombustible treatment. Wood, used in the interior and treated so that the beauty of the grain is brought out, is silken textured, satin surfaced, sympathetic to the hand and eye. Used with sensitive understanding of their inherent characteristics, the commonly available materials can be made to serve the needs of beauty as well as function and to elicit the desired emotional response.

Color. Space is the significant element, and, with its enclosing planes and forms, creates a place—a place that becomes a background for the users and their activities. The users are the active participants, the protagonists, who, with their necessary properties, provide the action and the color. It follows, then, that the background—the enclosing planes—be treated as background. Neutral colors, warm or cool, as the specific use or orientation of the space enclosed may determine, are the most desirable. The earth colors of brick and wood and lightly stained plaster are ideal. Expanses of bright-hued colors of high saturation are useful and often decorative in commercial establishments designed to catch the eye but in a treatment center or school are distracting, often garish, and in a short time become wearily tedious. A particular element or form, when function or delight requires, may be accented with brightly colored ceramic tiles or any other means of introducing a restrained amount of lively color.

THE PLANNING PROCESS

How do we apply this basic knowledge in planning a day treatment center? What are the steps to be followed and the areas to be considered each step of the way? The paragraphs that follow attempt to carry the reader through the process, first, by identifying the important features about day treatment that the architect needs to know, and second, by discussing the various elements involved in the architectural program.

Although it has many very special requirements not found in a typical elementary school, a center for emotionally disturbed children is essentially a school and will have most, if not all, of the functional elements found in the usual public school. Added to these are the special requirements of the therapeutic program. Just as therapeutic methods are integrated into the teaching, so must there be special architectural qualities integrated into the building, qualities that are articulated by means of form and materials.

Recommended Areas

A search of the literature has uncovered very little useful information concerning space requirements for the type of treatment center that is the present subject, although information on public schools abounds. In my architectural practice, I was first confronted with this question in 1958 when I was commissioned to design Wallace Village for Children, Broomfield, Colorado, a residential treatment center for children with organically based learning problems. Subsequently, I designed The Day Care Center, University of Colorado Health Sciences Center, a day treatment center for emotionally disturbed children and other similar institutions, such as the Rene Spitz Children's Division of the Fort Logan Mental Health Center.

For these facilities, area determinations were made by logical derivation from public school standards, anthropometric data, and extensive consultation with clients on the activities that would take place in the various spaces.

The recommended areas in the following paragraphs derive from the original determinations, revised where many years of use indicated the desirability or need for revision. Similarly, the assumptions leading to the estimate of the optimum number of children for which the building should be designed were based on the experience of these centers.

The Architectural Program

The preparation of a formal document, the architectural program, designed to define and organize the needs of the users, is the necessary beginning of the project. A complete architectural program should make clear the intended use of the facility, describing the therapeutic and educational aims and methods.

Goals of Day Treatment. At its inception in the early 1940s, day treatment was seen as a treatment modality more closely approximating a normal environment for moderately and severely emotionally handicapped children (Zimet & Farley, 1985). Its further growth and development coincided with the movement, generally, toward the deinstitutionalization of emotionally handicapped persons and the attempt to create a new set of attitudes toward the "mentally ill." It was, and continues to this day, to be conceived of as a setting that provides a total therapeutic environment without taking these children out of their homes and separating them from their families and neighborhoods, evenings, nights, and weekends. The day treatment facility involves children in interaction with a multidisciplinary staff 6 to 8 hours each day, 5 days a week, year around, and a minimum of 1 hour once-a-week therapeutic contact with families. It is a place where habilitative and rehabilitative interventions focus on all domains of the children's lives: the affective, relational, social, and educational. In effect, this total therapeutic program is made up of several definable components, such as a comprehensive therapeutic school program and individual, group, and family psychotherapy for children, as well as a therapeutic and consultative program for parents and families.

Other Objectives. Day treatment facilities are located in a variety of different settings. Most are found within larger institutional complexes such as the campuses of university medical centers, in general or psychiatric hospitals and clinics, and in state or county school systems. In such cases, they are likely to adopt the broad goals of their hosts along with the specific goals and objectives of a day treatment program. For example, although service and staff development may be the primary goals of most day treatment programs, additional goals would include training and research—the training of mental health professionals such as psychiatrists, psychiatric nurses, psychologists, social workers, and teachers, and the carrying out of research to further our knowledge about emotionally handicapped children and their families and about the efficacy of day treatment. The adoption of these objectives has an impact on planning for space and equipment needs.

The Number of Children and Staff. The architectural program should state the total number of children to be served, their age range, the proposed child to teacher ratio and class size, the number of professional and support people needed to staff the center and, when applicable, the number of trainees and research staff and the space they need. In order to clarify day-to-day activities, it is helpful to include a schedule of activities for a typical week.

The first question that must be dealt with in preparing the architectural program is the number of children for whom the project is to be designed. The question of the optimum number does not seem to have been addressed at any time; it is, however, of primary importance in planning a new building and, short of an arbitrary determination, the number must be deduced from experiential information.

Following are some empirical deductions derived from the experience of one center (The Day Care Center, University of Colorado Health Sciences Center), all of which lead to a reasonably conclusive determination for planning purposes (G. K. Farley, personal communication, February 10, 1987).

1. It has become apparent that six is the largest number of children that one teacher and one aid can adequately control and still maintain high-quality educational standards.
2. The ratio of professional staff members (teachers, psychiatrists, psychologists, social workers) is something in excess of three to every four children.
3. At least one professional staff member should know as much as can be known about at least one child.
4. The emotionally disturbed child must be encouraged to feel a part of the group and be able to know and be friends with every other member of the group. The child must not be overwhelmed by numbers.
5. To provide space to allow these conditions to take place, the area of the building must be on the order of 600 square feet per child, about 10 times that required for the typical public elementary school.

The inferential conclusion seems to indicate a maximum enrollment of 25 children. The discussion of functional requirements that follows is based on that number.

Constraints. The program is also concerned with constraints: the area and conformation of the site, geometry, building and zoning ordinances, limitation of budget and time, and other possible constraints.

Institutional Setting. The larger institutional setting within which the day treatment center might function has a direct bearing in many ways on the planning of the center: policies governing construction procedures, capital and operating budgeting systems, land use, personnel, and similar matters, all of which must be included in the program, in greater or lesser detail, depending upon applicability. Also to be included are the amounts and kinds of services the institution can provide, services such as central heating and cooling systems, general maintenance and housekeeping, central supplies, and the like.

Space, Quality, Cost. Notice must be taken of the important ratio of space, quality, and cost because that ratio will govern the design and construction of the center. It is axiomatic that these factors be placed in balance to avoid a frustrating experience when construction bids are opened. In applying the "Space × Quality = Cost" formula, only two of the three factors can be fixed by the center, the architect must be allowed to vary the third. If space and cost are rigid requirements, the only variable is quality of materials and construction. Obviously, the space required to carry out the therapeutic programs is essential and unless appropriate materials, equipment, and finishes are used, maintenance and operational costs may be excessively burdensome. Cheap and inadequate facilities save little initially and, for the long run, are, indeed, poor investments and permanent handicaps to the educational and therapeutic processes.

Cost is probably the most decisive limiting factor, rather than the number of children who might be treated. The previously listed assumptions demonstrate quite clearly that the program is expensive both in initial capital expenditure and in operating cost, although less costly than alternative inpatient or residential care. In the long run, undoubtedly it is less costly than the rehabilitation or support of broken lives at a later time. Unlike the public school, little or no economic advantage can be gained by increasing the scale because the center, to conform with the conditions listed, would necessarily have to be composed of several self-contained, discrete units, with central administration and large-scale purchasing the only possible source of financial advantage.

At this stage of the project, it is quite difficult to make an accurate cost estimate. Reliance must be placed on the cost of recently completed projects of a similar nature. Adjustments must be made for inflation, size and quality differences, location, local economic conditions at the time the completed building was bid, and predictions of what these conditions might be when the proposed building will be put out for bids. The budget should include a reasonable contingent amount. As the design process progresses, updated estimates must be made based on increasing amounts of information generated by the advancing studies, and necessary adjustments made so as to maintain the space, quality, and cost balance.

Safety Requirements. Schools, by the nature of their occupancy and use, require higher standards of safety than many other occupancy types. Provisions for life safety have the highest priority and can affect the entire design in plan, construction, and the choice of materials. All phases of safety and health become pervasive program elements that can add, unavoidably, to their complexity and cost. For this reason, among others, the single-story building is preferable. Among those reasons is the necessity for providing access to all parts of the building by physically handicapped people. This requirement can, of course, be met for buildings of two or more stories by the installation of elevators, thus adding to the cost of the building, as well as increasing maintenance costs.

Most building codes have specific requirements for school construction and, because conformance is mandatory, there is little need to do more than note that many code requirements are less demanding than good practice would ordinarily suggest. Because of the general characteristics of emotionally disturbed children, certain minimum code standards are inadequate. For example, The Uniform Building Code (The International Conference of Building Officials, 1985), used extensively in the western part of the country, requires doors to rooms having an occupancy load of 50 or more, to swing out in the direction of exit travel. The day treatment center classrooms have an occupancy load considerably less and would be exempt from the requirement, but for these children, in the event of an emergency, safe exiting demands that the doors swing in the direction of exit travel.

Site Selection

As noted earlier, very probably the center will be located within the boundaries of a larger institutional setting, in which case there will probably be little choice allowed in the selection of the site. If this is not the case, some basic particulars that should be considered in site selection are (a) present and future economic and social composition of the area; (b) integration with community planning and zoning requirements and limitations; (c) site characteristics that include percentage of usability for building, play areas, parking, and adequate landscaping, as well as soil conditions including height of water table, adjacent watersheds, and structural suitability; and (d) availability of utility services.

Urban Location. In a densely built, urban location, a site will often be quite small, offering little, if any, choice in orientation and severely limiting playground and garden areas. Undesirable as it may be, necessity may dictate a multilevel building, a much tighter plan, rooftop playgrounds, and potted plants.

> All places that the eye of heaven visits
> Are to a wise man ports and happy havens,
> Teach thy necessity to reason thus;
> There is no virtue like necessity.
>> Shakespeare, *King Richard II*,
>> Act I, Sc. 3, Line 275

Site Planning

Vehicular and pedestrian access, orientation, location of adjacent buildings, existing vegetation, drainage patterns, and utility service locations are the major determinants in planning the site. Some of these are discussed in detail next.

Vehicular and Pedestrian Access. Vehicular and pedestrian access and location of utilities connections to the mains will be the principal determinants of the building location. Because, in all probability, the site will be relatively small, its topography can be easily altered if necessary. Vehicular access, parking, and service must be separated from the play areas by physical barriers—the building, garden walls or fences—and, from the point of view of appearance, the service area and access should be visually isolated. Unless an institutional setting provides adequate parking areas for staff use, there should be provided one parking space for each staff member in addition to spaces for parents and other visitors. There should be a drop-off space at the entrance, so planned that the children can walk from car to entrance without crossing a traffic lane.

Climatic Considerations. As for a building of any occupancy, its location with respect to climate and latitude will affect the orientation, construction techniques, materials, and often the form. The arid and semiarid areas of the Southwest require different orientation than do humid areas in other parts of the country; the Northwest and the Great Lakes areas have many fewer sunlit days than the western mountain region and the Southwest. Current technology is capable of ameliorating the effect of the various climatic conditions, but it is usually less expensive in capital and operating costs to design the building taking advantage of the beneficial aspects of the climate and providing protection against the adverse. It is astonishing how often known climatic patterns are ignored and reliance placed wholly upon technology, sometimes with unfortunate results.

Generally, in the upper and middle latitudes of the United states, when the thermal component is considered, window walls are preferably southeast or south facing; southwest and west orientations are to be avoided whenever possible because those exposures receive excessive solar heat and north-facing windows are thermally vulnerable to cold, northerly storms.

Unfortunately, a building properly oriented to exploit the warmth of winter sunshine is not necessarily oriented to achieve optimum daylighting conditions; north light is probably the most desirable, providing a more nearly uniform light level with the least amount of glare. Careful balancing of the opposing factors, the use of insulating glass, roof overhangs, and other devices will mitigate the adverse effects and help resolve the paradox of the thermal, luminous elements.

Noise, Temperature, and Light. The physical aspects of the interior environment, those relating to the bodily senses of temperature, vision, and hearing, may be relatively well controlled by known engineering methods, but rational orientation and well-designed landscaping can be very effective in lessening the need for special construction methods or overly complicated mechanical systems and controls. For example, placing a noisy gym distant from quiet classrooms reduces the need for sound-attenuating materials. Admitting midday winter sun is desirable and, with the use of roof overhangs, summer sun can be blocked, but controlling the glare and heat of morning and afternoon sun when rooms are oriented to the east or west is considerably more difficult. When possible, windows in the east or west walls should be reduced to a minimum, if not omitted altogether. The use of roof overhangs has other advantages. They diffuse the light entering the building, creating a softer, pleasanter atmosphere. They protect the exterior walls, particularly in humid climates. Of possibly greater importance is the feeling of shelter they evoke, and, with the interior ceiling aligned with the exterior soffit and window heads raised to the same height, the sheltering effect is greatly enhanced.

Exterior Functional Requirements

Landscaping. In addition to rational orientation, well-designed landscaping can contribute to the operating efficiency and comfort of the building. Deciduous trees permit the winter sun to penetrate and provide shade from the heat of the summer sun; shrubs can be used effectively in combination with trees as windbreaks, the shrubs slowing the wind passing under the trees; and planting helps control dust, dirt, heat, glare, and surface drainage. In the selection of plant materials, it is desirable, whenever possible, to use those that are indigenous to the region and to supplement them with adapted exotic plants possessing characteristics not obtainable with local materials.

Playground. The main playground, preferably south facing and directly accessible from the playroom (gymnasium), should have an area of 500 to 600 square feet for each child and be separated by landscape features, a wall or fence, from a smaller area of approximately 300 square feet per child for the younger children. The ground should be reasonably level, well drained, and have the usual age-appropriate play equipment. Except for certain specific spaces, turf seems to be the most satisfactory surfacing material, although it does require considerable maintenance. Resilient paving is desirable at basketball practice goals, other apparatus areas, and for the use of wheeled toys for the younger children. Acceptable alternatives to resilient paving at playground equipment such as swings, slides, climbing gyms, and the like are tanbark, sand, and various types of synthetic surfacing materials. The larger playground, if situated in view of the classrooms, can be a distraction for those children not at play, and, consequently, it is desirable to locate it in a less visually accessible place. All the playgrounds should be enclosed by masonry walls or solid wood fences.

Outdoor Classroom. A desirable component that might be considered in site planning is the outdoor classroom, one of which might be planned immediately outside each classroom, and which could serve as a play space for the younger children. The inclusion of such space would provide a convenient location for gardening projects, salutary, and often quieting activities.

Building Materials

Resistive Properties. To the extent that a generalization can be made of the characteristics of emotionally disturbed children, those that can affect the design of a building are the limitations in their ability to tolerate frustration, the regulation of feelings, and reality testing. Many of these children are unable to contain strong feelings and often discharge them in an explosive, destructive way. Obviously, it is necessary to select building materials that will best resist impulsive behavior directed at the nonretaliative building.

Materials commonly used in the building industry having the necessary resistive properties are masonry, wood, and heavy gauge metal. Plaster can be damaged, but it is unlikely. Gypsum board, extensively used for wall and partition finish, cannot be recommended because it has little impact resistance, although it is easily repaired. Glass, within hitting or kicking distance, must be tempered or laminated; the latter is preferable because it will maintain integrity even though cracked. Prudence suggests its use throughout. Although putty is rarely used today to secure glass in its frame, it should be avoided because it is a prime target for fingernails, even for normal children. Replacement costs are reduced if windows and glazed doors are provided with muntins to reduce the size of individual panes. Doors should be solid core rather than hollow.

Floors, except possibly in the playroom (gymnasium), should be carpeted; although it is somewhat more difficult to clean when water-based paint is spilled, its advantages, including its sound-absorbing properties, are more than enough to balance. Playroom (gymnasium) floors are often maple, but a good grade of vinyl or rubber tile is a satisfactory economic substitute, and carpet is a good possibility with added acoustic qualities.

Thermostats and other controls must have tamperproof covers. Tables, seating two or more children, that are designed and built with solid panels separating knee space, will prevent kicking games. Doors that stick, hardware that is maladjusted or of poor quality, and equipment that does not operate or function smoothly and easily, increase frustration and exacerbate tendencies to violent behavior. High-quality maintenance is of very great importance.

Interior Functional Requirements

The Classroom. The core of the treatment center is the classroom that should be designed with an area of 85 to 100 square feet per child. The usual classroom fixtures should be installed: work counters as long as possible with cabinets below for storage of books, paper, maps, audiovisual equipment, and the like; a sink with bubbler installed at a convenient place; and a teacher's closet and filing cabinet. Classrooms for the younger children should have a two-fixture toilet room accessible directly from the classroom, and provision should be made in the classroom for coat and boot storage. Coat storage for the older children can be in the classroom or in the corridor immediately adjacent.

The area, as noted, of each classroom is sufficiently large to accommodate seat arrangements for any purpose and still allow adequate area for special projects and the necessary equipment such as aquaria, terraria, small animal cages, and so on. A useful element that might be included in the classroom is a small alcove—a sort of cave—where a child with a temporary onset of atavism or who feels his or her level of frustration rising, might go to get away from it all. Provision also must be made in all classrooms for darkening the room for audiovisual presentations.

It is important that the height of work surfaces and other fixtures be appropriate to the age group. This requirement may present some difficulties in the arts and crafts room, although it is probable that the younger children will do that work in their own classroom.

Observation Rooms. Observation rooms, each large enough to seat comfortably four or five adults, are essential for observation of each classroom, the arts room, and at least half the number of interview rooms. It is economically desirable to so organize the plan that one room can look into two or more rooms, but between the constraints of geometry and the necessity of having a maximum of chalk and tack boards, of having sufficient windows for adequate daylighting and the required book-shelving and storage cabinets, it becomes difficult to so arrange the plan. Videotaping and closed circuit, remote-controlled television are not adequate substitutes for direct observation. Videotaping will be done and is necessary for documentation, but the observation rooms are still necessary.

Arts and Crafts Room. An arts and crafts room, although not absolutely necessary, is highly desirable. The room provides space to expand this adjunct activity with all its necessary equipment and supplies and concentrates the disorder that usually accompanies painting, modeling, and other craftwork. The essential requirements are plenty of space, of work surface, of storage capacity, and of wall and shelf displays. Eight hundred to 900 square feet of floor area is adequate for five to eight children. Chalk boards are less needed than tack board space and can probably be omitted altogether, although it is desirable to have some.

Storage is needed for paper, paint, wood, and other crafts materials, and easels. Watertight and reasonably airtight bins for clay and cubicles for each child to store work in progress are necessary. There should be three or four sinks, one of which should be fitted with a solids interceptor. A small electric kiln should be installed.

An abundance of north daylight is desirable and, to save wall space for display and storage, can be supplied by a roof monitor or sawtooth type of skylight, with the glazed area north facing.

Child Psychotherapy Rooms. Child psychotherapy rooms have several functions, the principal use being for individual therapy, which use determines the size and the built-in fixtures it should have. A second and equally important use is as a secluded place to which a child, losing control, can immediately be taken for professional help in regaining composure. Because of this use, the rooms must be as close as possible to the classrooms. The rooms will also be used for parent and staff conferences involving a few people when it is more convenient than a staff office.

There should be one room for every 8 or 10 children; each should have an area of 125 to 150 square feet, a workcounter with sink and storage for paper, paint, and other play-therapy equipment, and chalk and tack boards. Partitions and ceiling should have a sound transmission class (STC) of 60 to 65 at least.

The Playroom. The playroom, a small gymnasium, should have an area of 1,500 to 2,000 square feet. The addition of a small stage with proscenium, stage curtain, cyclorama, and adequate stage lighting increases its usefulness and provides a setting for children's plays and formal assemblies. Basketball goals should be installed, as well as floor inserts to receive volleyball net and other apparatus supports. Adequate storage is required for indoor and outdoor play equipment and folding or stacking chairs. If the room is daylighted, the windows should be clerestory with sills at least 7 feet above the floor and equipped with woven wire guards and light-tight blinds. The playroom should open directly onto the larger playground.

The Lunchroom. With the addition of wall shelves, the lunchroom can also serve as the library, an informal, small collection of children's books. The room can also serve as a conference room. It should look out on and have access to a playground or small garden, with windows and doors south facing. The required area is 15 to 17 square feet for each sitting, with tables seating three to four children and two adults. The floor should be carpeted and the finishes, wherever possible, should be of sound-absorbing materials to reduce the noise level.

Because the menu is simple and everyone is served the same lunch, the serving counter need only be a 4-to-6-feet-wide pass window at kitchen-counter level and should have a built-in steam table; a second window, 3 to 4 feet wide, adjacent to the dishwasher, can receive the soiled dishes.

The Kitchen. The kitchen is a rather important place, particularly if the cook enjoys baking cookies and having children underfoot. The space required is about 250 square feet and should be planned in much the same way as a large residential kitchen. Generally, high-quality, heavy-duty, domestic appliances serve adequately and will give many years of trouble-free use. Storage requirements, refrigerated and dry, depend in great part on purchasing policies.

Offices for Professional and Support Staff. An office, 100 to 150 square feet in area, should be planned for each member of the professional staff; if a training program is included, a single room with an area of 40 to 50 square feet per person will serve as an office for the trainees. It is desirable to have a conference room large enough to seat the entire staff, although the lunch room can serve that purpose; if a conference room is included, 25 square feet per person should be allowed. Offices for the secretarial pool should have adequate record and office supply storage and adequate areas to house electronic office equipment, such as computers, printers, and copiers. The usual reception and waiting room, staff lounge, toilet rooms, mechanical equipment, and housekeeping spaces complete the list of room requirements. The selection of mechanical and electrical systems should be made before the area of the space to house the equipment is finally determined; inadequate space makes servicing difficult, and, consequently, leads to a tendency on the part of maintenance people to shirk routine servicing.

General Locations. Preferably, all the functional elements should be on the ground floor, although mechanical equipment and housekeeping stores are better located in a basement, with the mechanical equipment in a sound-isolated space. The classrooms, arts and crafts rooms, and the child psychotherapy rooms should be grouped and as proximate as possible. For greater efficiency and comfort of the professional staff, their offices should be located reasonably close to the classrooms; however, if the area of the site is severely limited, these offices, that of the trainees, staff lounge, and toilet rooms can be located on a second floor. Playroom (gymnasium), lunchroom, and kitchen should be so located that their noisy activities will not disturb the relative quiet of the classrooms, staff offices, and conference room.

Flexibility and Planning for Change

Science and technology are continually creating new ideas, new methods, new products that, in turn, engender changes in the way we do whatever we do. We have learned that we must plan into our buildings a certain amount of flexibility, the amount determined in great part by the use to which the building will be put. It is almost impossible to predict the kind and degree of change that may take place in the future, but we know that growth is almost inevitable despite initial growth-limiting policy. These limits may be, and often are, altered for a variety of reasons. We know that the need to experiment to achieve better results is always with us. Provision for future additions, the use of movable partitions and fixtures of all sorts can allow for these possible eventualities.

The Public School Experience. In considering the extent of flexibility desirable in a day treatment center, a brief review of the experience of the public school system in the past forty years will be useful. It is well known that at the end of World War II, the country's school systems were faced with large and rapidly growing enrollments and a severe teacher shortage (Alvey, 1984). Concurrently, innovative teaching methods were instituted, some derived from armed services training experiences, others devised to mitigate the shortage of qualified teachers (Alvey, 1984). Included in the list of innovations were team teaching, audiovisual and electronic teaching devices, ungraded and independent study programs, and the like. The traditional closed classroom was ill-suited for these methods and was replaced by the open-plan concept—very large open spaces divided only by movable partitions and wheeled cabinets. This afforded the desired flexibility, but there were several serious faults, not the least being acoustic problems. More recently, the school systems appear to be seeking a middle ground, providing fixed rooms of various sizes, with movable partitions in the larger ones, thus allowing some degree of flexible use.

In the Day Treatment Center. There are two factors acting together that reduce or eliminate the need for such devices. The first is the very high ratio of professional staff to pupil; although not all staff members are teachers, the therapeutic and educational processes are so integrated that the relationship of staff to pupil is almost one to one. The second factor is the ratio of building area to pupil, a ratio of approximately 10 times that of the public school. Considering these factors and with the added advantage of having spaces available for several purposes, varying in size from 10 feet by 15 feet to classroom size, the flexibility is built in, and it seems unnecessary to provide additional devices such as movable partitions. The plan, however, should be so organized that future additions for growth or change of the program are possible.

A caveat when considering the use or incorporation of flexible devices: If flexibility is carried to an extreme, or even part way there, it will almost inevitably result in a loss of character—a loss of those environmental qualities that affect feelings and behavior. No matter how skillfully the elements are designed, the very geometry of the three-dimensional space necessarily becomes uniform and bland; fenestration must be uniform, ceilings of a uniform height, and every element so arranged that all fit anywhere. The feeling of permanence, with the security that these special children need, is lost.

CONCLUSION

Essentially, a building to house a treatment center must be so designed that emotionally disturbed children can feel it to be a haven of security, a place that carries no hint of threat, that welcomes and encourages. It should surround the children with beauty and invite them to take pleasure in learning, and above all, be sheltering.

REFERENCES

Alvey, E., Jr. (1984). Elementary education. In D. Holland (Ed.), *The Encyclopedia Americana* (Vol. 9. pp. 671–672). Danbury, CT: Grolier, Inc.

International Conference of Building Officials. (1985). *The Uniform Building Code.* Whittier, CA: International Conference of Building Officials.

Zimet, S. G., & Farley, G. K. (1985). Day treatment for children in the United States. *Journal of the American Academy of Child Psychiatry, 24,* 732–738.

II

Program Models

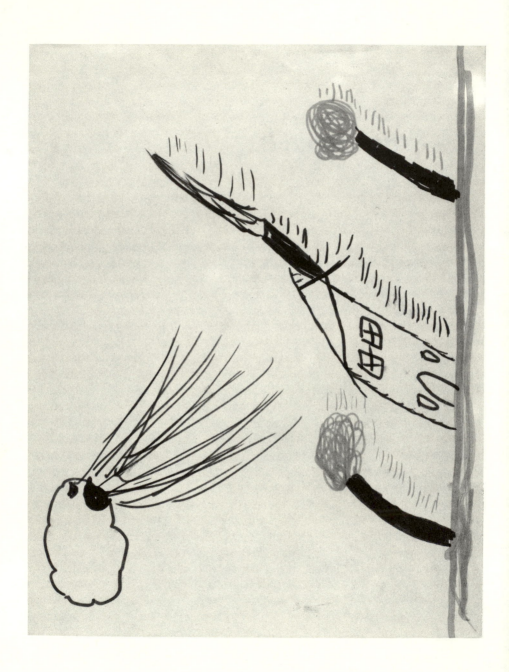

In this part, which includes Chapters 4 through 9, a variety of program models is presented. Because no form of day psychiatric treatment has clearly demonstrated superior efficacy to another, it is entirely reasonable that we should present a number of apparently competing but in truth complementary models. In fact, few settings blindly employ a single, narrowly defined model. Settings that consider themselves behavioral almost always consider biological, sociocultural, and psychodynamic contributors to their children's and families' problems. Some of these models, such as the psychodynamic model, grow from theoretical considerations, whereas others, such as the model for disadvantaged children or the model for afterschool day treatment, attempt to address the needs of particular populations.

In Chapter 4, Gaston Blom, a child, adolescent, and adult psychiatrist and psychoanalyst, treats us to a description of a relatively new perspective in the treatment of children with serious emotional disturbances. He makes cogent criticisms of the squandering of scarce resources on ineffective traditional treatments and makes a convincing case that the rehabilitation perspective offers new hope to a poorly treated population.

In Chapter 5, Laurel Kiser and David Pruitt describe the theoretical basis for the program discussed in Chapter 2. They show us how the data from a wide variety of sources are capably integrated into a comprehensive and comprehensible treatment plan.

Robert Lyman and Steven Prentice-Dunn, both clinical child psychologists, describe in Chapter 6 a carefully thought out and well-documented program based on behavioral principles. Of all treatment methods, behavioral treatments are perhaps best at generating usable data, and in this chapter, the authors illustrate how the data derived from such a program can lead to validation of their treatment efforts.

In Chapter 7, Janet Newman, a psychoanalyst and child psychiatrist and the director of a day treatment program for many years, thoroughly and sensitively leads us through the remarkable depth work done by a psychodynamically oriented program. She shows how information from a child's life and emotional–developmental history can be used both in individual child psychotherapy and in the milieu treatment.

Stewart Gabel, Mark Finn, and Robert Catenaccio, in Chapter 8, discuss a program that offers treatment to a difficult and underserved population. Gabel, a pediatrician and child psychiatrist, Finn, a psychologist, and Catenaccio, a child psychiatrist, offer an open and honest discussion of their creative attempts to involve parents in their treatment efforts and the results of these efforts.

Ellie Sternquist, a clinical child psychologist, tells us in Chapter 9 of a remarkable adaptation to the needs of the community and describes an afterschool day treatment program that was funded on a shoestring and continues to serve community needs in an important way. This program can be thought of as a model for several different agencies working together to provide services for children.

4

Developmental Rehabilitation Perspectives in the Day Treatment of Children with Serious Emotional Disorders

GASTON E. BLOM

INTRODUCTION

The importance of a developmental rehabilitation perspective in clinical and educational programs for seriously emotionally disturbed children has evolved from the author's 40 years of professional experience in university and community settings. The purpose of this chapter is to present the rationale for this approach in working with emotionally disturbed children in general, and, especially, in working with those where long-term conventional treatments have been unsuccessful.

First, a group of adolescents will be described who were seen in psychiatric consultation during a period of 4 years. They represent a sample of young people with chronic, severe emotional disturbances who moved through conventional service systems during early childhood to later adolescence without a resolution of past or present problems.

GASTON E. BLOM • South Shore Mental Health Center, 77 Parking Way, Quincy, Massachusetts 02169.

65

Then, in the pages of the chapter that follow, a number of perspectives will be discussed that relate to developmental rehabilitation as a model for interventions. These perspectives include the prevalence and social status of children with emotional disorders; the stigmatization that severely emotionally disturbed children and youth face in their community and from human service professionals; the availability and quality of services to treat such disorders; the short- and long-term effectiveness of conventional treatment and special education services; and a developmental rehabilitation model and its application to chronically emotionally disturbed children and youth.

CLINICAL ASPECTS OF CHRONICITY

Clinical illustrations of chronicity and the disabling and handicapping consequences of serious emotional disturbance most readily come from adolescent development. At this age, these phenomena become more manifest, especially as adaptation expectations increase. One can look at clinical cases retrospectively to identify opportunities that existed earlier in development where the repetitive and unresponsive cycle of traditional treatment and educational approaches could have been modified. At other times, clinical and educational decisions can be seen in hindsight as intensifying but continuing what had not been successful before.

Severe emotional disturbance, as it becomes chronic, characteristically involves many service systems and absorbs a great deal of professional time and resources. At the point of established chronicity, the disabling consequences of the severe impairment to the individual and the handicapping results in adaptive environmental functioning become more important than the disturbance itself (World Health Organization, 1980). Prior to the turning point of established chronicity, consequences of impairment can already be identified. Eventually, the disturbance may no longer respond to remediation, and primary goals of treatment and education become illusory.

Regarding severely emotionally disturbed children, Lourie and Katz-Leavy (1986) point to the limited value of diagnosis and the use of the medical treatment model. The medical model does not relate to issues of severity and chronicity or to the issue that many of these children will need services in adult life. Furthermore, the concept of chronicity is alien to child mental health and special education thinking. It implies negativity and hopeless situations about which nothing can be done within the parameters of those models. On the other hand, the concepts of consequences of chronic disorder in terms of disability and handicap point to rehabilitation assessment of the individual and his/her environment that can generate realistic intervention options (Wright, 1983).

A description of a group of seven adolescents who were referred for emergency psychiatric outpatient consultation at a community mental health center over a 6-month period demonstrates the chronicity, disability, and handicap issues. These seven young people were in middle to late adolescence. Problem behaviors, DSM-III diagnoses (American Psychiatric Association, 1981), treatment placements, and other demographic information may be seen in Table 1.

The case records of all seven adolescents showed that a variety of treatment and educational/remedial interventions had been tried and that numerous and repeated extensive diagnostic evaluations had been done at university tertiary-care facilities. These evaluations provided extensive information on their disorders and impairments. Also impressive was the continued recommendation of similar treatments and remediations with only slight alterations. Yet over time, more restrictive placements were advised. In addition, many service agencies became involved in treatment, and sometimes the network of agencies acted in strikingly dysfunctional and fragmented ways similar to the dysfunction of the families of the adolescents.

This group of seven adolescents meet each of the criteria for severe emotional disturbance as defined by Lourie and Katz-Leavy (1986): (a) mental illness as defined by some classification system, (b) marked family dysfunction, (c) substantial functional limitations in major life activities, (d) severe disability of long duration, and (e) involvement with many human service agencies.

THE PREVALENCE AND SOCIAL STATUS OF SEVERELY EMOTIONALLY DISTURBED CHILDREN

Prevalence

Studies on emotional disturbance in children in the United States estimate the prevalence to be approximately 11.8% of the general child population, or 7.3 million (Gould, Wunsch-Hitzig, & Dohrenwend, 1981). The proportion identified as severely emotionally disturbed includes 5% of that number or 300,000 children (American Academy of Child Psychiatry, 1983; Knitzer & Olson, 1982; Lourie & Katz-Leavy, 1986).

Table 1. Descriptive Characteristics of Seven Seriously Disturbed Adolescents

Age	17.09	17.0	16.0	17.0	16.0	15.5	15.5
Gender	F	F	F	M	M	M	M
Diagnosis	Dysthymic disorder	Manic depressive illness	Reactive psychosis	Conduct disorder	Dysthymic disorder	Paranoid schizophrenia	Conduct disorder
Behaviors							
Alcohol and drugs	X	X	X	X	X	X	X
Physically abusive		X		X	X	X	X
Suicidal	X	X	X		X	X	
Runs away	X	X	X	X		X	X
Treatments							
Psychiatric hospitalizations	2 times	2 times	4 times	Detention center	1 time	1 time	2 times
Residential placement	Recommended	2 years	4 years	Recommended	2 years	Recommended	2 years
Psychoactive meds	X	X	X	Recommended	X	X	X
Special education	1st grade LD to EBD	Elementary EBD	1st grade LD to EBD	Elementary EBD-dropout	1st grade LD to EBD	1st grade LD to EBD	2nd grade EBD

Note. LD = learning disability; EBD = emotional and behavioral disorder; F = female; M = male; X = characteristic present.

Social Attitudes and Stigmatization

Seriously emotionally disturbed children and their families are probably more stigmatized than any other disabled group (Tringo, 1972). Furthermore, these children are disturbing to schools and communities, as well as to social agencies and to professionals who serve them (Goffman, 1963). They have few advocates and are not usually objects of charity or sympathy. In fact, most professionals avoid treating or otherwise addressing their needs and prefer to devote their time to "more treatable" patients with minor problems. Some time ago this was referred to as "rejection by the learned" (Joint Commission on Mental Health of Children, 1969).

A recent report on the attitudes of child psychiatrists toward their work indicates that their personal satisfactions were correlated with the degree of psychological disturbance in the patients they treated. Positive attitudes were associated with treating children having moderate disturbance, physical disabilities, learning disabilities, and situations of acute crisis. Negative attitudes were associated with severe psychiatric disturbance, abuse, delinquency, and retardation. These child psychiatrists also indicated a preference to decrease further their professional work level with child abuse, delinquency, and mental retardation (American Academy of Child Psychiatry, 1983).

Words, images, and labels also represent ways in which stigma is communicated and absorbed. *Crazy, psycho, weirdo, mental,* and *retard* are some of the more common labels assigned to emotionally disturbed children in special classes. Children perceive the concept, emotional disturbance, more negatively than other disabilities. When the behaviors of disturbed children are labeled as deviant, normal children like them less (Chiba, 1984).

In response to such concerns, an amendment to the Education of Handicapped Children's Act was considered in 1983 to change the terminology from "seriously emotionally disturbed" to "behaviorally disordered." A study contracted by the Department of Education to investigate this issue concluded that a change in terminology would have little or no positive impact on service delivery. However, in states where the term *emotionally disturbed* was used, many psychologists and parents were reluctant to assign this label because of its potentially stigmatizing effect. In other states where *behaviorally disordered* was employed, the opinion was often expressed that this was an educational rather than a medical term. This change made it preferable to *emotionally disturbed,* which was negatively associated with a medical psychiatric problem (National Association of State Directors of Special Education, 1985).

CRITIQUE OF CURRENT EDUCATIONAL AND CLINICAL SERVICES

Availability and Quality of Services

Two-thirds of severely disturbed children have no specific services available to meet their particular needs (Knitzer & Olson, 1982). In fact, mental health services are more likely to be provided children with less serious disorders (Pfeiffer, 1984). Services such as a coordinated system of support, advocacy networks for parents, and community-based services are lacking. Emergency services, therapeutic foster care, home care, and day psychiatric treatment are also not available. The shortcomings of policy and practice with severely emotionally disturbed children are particularly troublesome, because evidence indicates that such children remain chronically disturbed throughout childhood and adolescence into adult life (Lourie & Katz-Leavy, 1986).

Not only is the majority of severely disturbed children underserved, but among the one-third for whom services are available, a significant proportion are being poorly served. There are ample examples for this assertion. The classification of exceptional children project indicates that children, classified as delinquent or in need of supervision, often receive harsher treatment than would an adult with the same offense. Diagnostic evaluations of emotionally disturbed children, repeatedly done, often became ends in themselves rather than a means to appropriate services (Hobbs, Egerton, & Matheny, 1975).

A lack of interdisciplinary and interagency collaboration and community planning in service delivery also is seen as contributing to poor quality care. The delivery of appropriate services suffers when collaboration is limited or nonexistent. This is particularly true with seriously disturbed children where troubled systems confound the problems of troubled children.

Effectiveness of Special Education Services

In recent years, statewide follow-up data have been reported on secondary special education programs in all disability categories from Colorado (Mithaug, Horiuchi, & Fanning, 1985), Oregon (Halpern, 1985), Vermont (Hasazi, Gordon, & Roe, 1985), Virginia (Wehman, Kregel, & Barcus, 1985), and Washington State (Edgar, 1985; Maddox, Edgar, & Levine, 1984). There are limitations to these studies: (a)

Findings are not always analyzed separately for different disability groups and according to severity of disability; and (b) samples do not include sufficient numbers of emotionally disturbed children in proportion to their actual prevalence. Nevertheless, some interesting findings and implications emerge when looking at these studies as a group. These include the high incidence of school dropouts, unemployment, and a limited range of interpersonal relationships other than family.

The work status of graduates of special education programs averaged 69% employment, but often graduates worked only part time and earned less than minimum wage. Differences in employment were noted for some disability groups, such as 64% for behaviorally disordered and 38% for mildly retarded. Favorable factors associated with employment included mainstreaming with resource room assignments instead of segregated placements, experience with summer and part-time schoolyear jobs, and graduation versus leaving and/or dropping out of special programs. In addition, many of these graduates did not obtain further educational or technical training (50%), had not used vocational rehabilitation services (63%), had not contacted state employment services (65%), or did not enroll in mental health service programs for the developmentally disabled adults (96%).

Other findings indicated that 64% were still living at home with parents or guardians 4 years after graduation. Most of them had no or few friends outside the family. The studies indicate that features characterizing this group, such as family dependence, financial instability, and lack of postgraduate training and services, had not changed appreciably over the years from 1978 to 1983, even with the advent of PL 94-142.

These studies also pointed out the discrepancy between what teachers and administrators claimed was available for students and what parents and their children perceived as being available to them. Less than 50% of the parents thought their children received instruction in vocational preparation, functional academics, and community living skills. Two-thirds of the graduates believed that secondary education should have prepared them more fully for independent living, community participation, and job knowledge and selection.

The findings from outcome studies of secondary special education students underline the importance of transitional services to prepare young people for adult living. Only in more recent years has the need for transitional programs and planning been recognized. It is estimated that 300,000 students leave special education each year and that many of them become dependent members of the community (*Federal Register,* 1984).

Potential dropouts often find vocational education is a powerful incentive to remain in school and to find a future direction in work. Therefore, attempts were made to revise statutes in the 1984 Vocational Educational Act Extension by allocating a higher percentage of funds to special needs groups, promoting easier access to vocational education, improving the quality of programming for handicapped youth, and increasing collaboration with nonschool agencies (Lotto, 1985).

Effectiveness of Mental Health Services

It is difficult to find information and discourse in the mental health literature on the outcome and evaluation of treated emotionally disturbed children and adolescents. Public and private mental health, as systems, are less open to public examination than special education. There is a resistance to evaluate and compare treatment approaches and, in particular, to report on their long- and short-term effectiveness. Some of this reluctance stems from methodological problems inherent in clinical research, the cost in time and money to carry out these studies, as well as a naive optimism that good intentions are rewarded by good outcomes. Some relevant studies are summarized next.

Inpatient and Residential Treatment. Follow-up studies on emotionally disturbed children and adolescents that do exist point to the frequent persistence of symptoms into adult life, particularly with conduct disturbances (Shaffer, 1984). Lewis, Shanok, Klatskin, and Osborne (1980) reported a follow-up study of 51 children who had received 2 years of what appeared to be beneficial residential treatment. Two years later, two-thirds of this group were considered to have a poor outcome as measured by subsequent psychopathological and social adjustment indicators. The good-outcome group differed in being younger at the time of admission and follow-up and in showing more psychotic symptoms; in other dimensions the good and poor-outcome groups were similar.

Rutter (1983) reports the rapidity with which the positive effects of residential treatment may be undone. This phenomenon points to the importance of transitional programs from residential and inpatient settings to less restrictive ones. Because 15,000 children are estimated to be in residential treatment at any time (Blotcky, Dimperio, &

Gossett, 1984), the need for further outcome studies on residential treatment and psychiatric hospitalization is apparent.

Most follow-up reports on severely disturbed children who have been hospitalized are retrospective rather than prospective. These reports focus on factors associated with more favorable and less favorable outcomes (Blotcky, Dimperio, & Gossett, 1984; Gossett, Lewis, & Barnhart, 1983). Factors found to be associated with more favorable outcomes include less severe psychopathology, higher measured intelligence, and younger chronological age. Factors associated with less favorable outcomes were organic neurological dysfunction, multiple home placements, and parents with legal conflicts. The influence on outcome by such factors as frequency of treatment contacts, medication, length of hospital stay, and family cooperation was not found to be significant.

Day Psychiatric Treatment. Day psychiatric treatment for children with moderate to severe emotional disturbances has been proposed as a cost-effective alternative to inpatient hospitalization and residential treatment (Baenen, Stephens, & Glenwick, 1986; Gabel & Finn, 1986; Zimet & Farley, 1985). Yet, evidence on the effectiveness of day treatment is very sparse. There are no controlled studies comparing day treatment with other forms of intensive treatment such as inpatient care. There are some claims that severely disturbed children benefit from day treatment and make cognitive, academic, and behavioral–social gains that are fairly well maintained (Blom, Farley, & Ekanger, 1973; Zimet *et al.*, 1980). No comparison groups were utilized in these studies. Some studies have been done relating patient factors to outcome (Prentice-Dunn, Wilson, & Lyman, 1981). There is some suggestive evidence that children who are treated at an earlier age and whose families are more involved in treatment have more favorable outcomes (Gabel & Finn, 1986).

Attitudes toward Treatment. Although the identification and measurement of therapists' influence on children are difficult to determine, the finding that many children regularly say they do not like their therapists is a provocative one (Shaffer, 1984). The corollary is that many children in treatment may have little understanding of what therapy is about. Such factors probably influence dropout rates and may effect other outcome measures. Gracula, Rosenthal, Curtiss, and Marohn (1984) have studied the influences of coercive referral, internalizing or externalizing symptoms, ethnicity, social class, denial of a problem, and therapist characteristics on staying in treatment. Although only a small percentage of their adolescent sample stayed in treatment a significant amount of time, favorable influences noted included Caucasian ethnicity, upper-class membership, noncoercive referral, problem acceptance, and surprisingly, externalizing symptoms.

A DEVELOPMENTAL REHABILITATION PERSPECTIVE

The implications from the reports reviewed for seriously emotionally disturbed children and adolescents lead directly to the rehabilitation model proposed here. First, curricula must be designed for training independent living skills at all developmental age levels. Second, children and adolescents, with their parents, need to anticipate and prepare for coping with the transition points in their lives. Third, children and adolescents should be exposed to natural work situations and to a range of realistic vocational possibilities and opportunities. Fourth, career components should be made part of individual educational plans. Fifth, interagency agreements need to be established for transition periods, in particular, from adolescent to adult-oriented human services. Sixth, appropriate modifications of home, school, and work environments need to be made.

Application of a Physical Disability Model to Psychiatric Disorders

Anthony, Cohen, and Cohen (1983) and Falloon and others (*Rehab Brief,* 1983) have applied a physical disability rehabilitation model to severe psychiatric/psychological disorders of adults with some success. This model emphasizes skills training and support networks for living, learning, and working within practical functional social contexts. Treatments such as individual therapy, family treatment, and medication are recognized but receive less primary attention. These authors are of the opinion that psychiatric diagnosis does not specify how to intervene nor is it strongly related to outcome. Skill acquisitions rather than symptom reduction appear more related to positive outcomes. A training approach is advocated consisting of telling, showing, and practicing concrete skills in a number of life function domains—physical, emotional, and intellectual. The physical domain includes hygiene, cooking, recreation, transportation, body fitness, and work. The emotional domain refers to satisfactions, rewards, self-control, socialization, problem solving, and job seeking. The intellectual domain includes money management and functional computation and language skills.

The application of social skills training to adult chronic psychiatric patients has been reviewed by Brady (1984a,b). Skills for effective instrumental goals are presented along with inventories available for their assessment. Treatment approaches of instruction, modeling, rehearsal, feedback, reinforcement, homework, and generalization steps are addressed. Although these approaches are not always successful, they point to the needs of patients and families for coping skills and everyday living abilities that can be taught, rehearsed, and practiced.

Families of patients need to have their concerns and coping skills recognized. A rehabilitation diagnosis is developed from assessments of individual life skills and problems and his/her environments that impede or facilitate adaptation. These assessments become the basis for a specific individual rehabilitation plan. Interventions should obtain ongoing patient agreement, understanding, and involvement in each step of the program.

Transitions in the Life Span

Attention to significant transition points throughout the life span should be included in any rehabilitation program for children and adolescents. Models for older adolescents and adults have been proposed by Will (1984a,b) and by Halpern (1985). Transitions represent times of (a) special needs for security and structure, (b) particular biopsychosocial developmental stress, (c) opportunities for adaptation and progression, and (d) risks for maladaptation and regression. Examples of transitions for the impaired or unimpaired person would include change in status from a one-child family to a two-child family; unemployment of a parent; starting school for the first time; progressing to different levels of school later on; beginning employment; marriage; and divorce. For severely emotionally disabled persons, transitions might include moving from a more segregated environment, such as an institution or residential treatment center, to a more integrated mainstream placement at home and in a public school classroom.

Community Locus

The rehabilitation perspective emphasizes the importance of community adjustment in the areas of work, social networks, and independent living. Developmental transitions provide opportunities for rehabilitation perspectives to be employed by professionals in special education and mental health. In addition, within the rehabilitation approach, the sociological notions of stigmatization and its consequences are dealt with as a reality (Safilios-Rothschild, 1970).

Social Networks and Their Assessment

What is also proposed is an identification and modification of environmental components of seriously emotionally disturbed children who are in the process of development and who are realistically dependent on their environments. Disturbed children are particularly influenced by the many environmental contexts in which they live, such as home, school, and community (Hobbs, 1982). All children need support networks of caring, guiding, and protecting environments. Disturbed children's needs are all the more compelling and require environmental interventions for support, maintenance, and corrective influence. These environments should be assessed as part of program planning and intervention (Bronfenbrenner, 1979).

However, as Blom, Lininger, and Charlesworth (1987) indicate, the current state of ecological assessment is more an orientation than a methodology. There is continued reliance on traditional procedures of rating scales, tests, and interviews independent of social contexts for emotionally disturbed children. Results from these measures are not readily translated into intervention strategies within the natural environments of the child.

Despite these measurement limitations, an ecological view can be borrowed from the physical disability rehabilitation model. Assistance to parents can be modeled on the types of responses and reactions that parents have toward a physically disabled child. These include issues such as mourning the loss of the idealized child and lowered self-esteem resulting from perceived parental failures. In addition, the many ongoing stress issues of having a seriously disturbed child need to be addressed, such as the increased demands on parents' time, energy, and finances; pressures from work; and problems in home management and control (Blom, 1982). Parents have greater needs for concrete management suggestions than for psychodynamic understanding of behaviors and family conflicts.

Skills in Dealing with the World

As in the physical disability rehabilitation model, disturbed children need to be taught skills that directly relate to self-care, independent living, and vocational preparation. Emotionally disturbed children should be prepared to face and deal with stigma and negative social attitudes from the ablebodied and ableminded worlds. They also need professionals, enlightened citizens, and parents as advocates in their behalf. These children and adolescents should participate more fully and appropriately in the decision-making processes that directly affect them (Gillespie & Turnbull, 1983). These processes include aspects of their education, placement, treatment, training, and rehabilitation.

Comparisons of Three Human Service Systems

Table 2 contrasts the three approaches of rehabilitation, teaching, and treatment to emotional disturbance in the areas of goals, focus, assumptions, and activities. Within these services a developmental view is often limited. Special education lacks a future perspective and tends to focus on skills of the present. Treatment of adults does not sufficiently consider their childhood pasts, whereas treat-

Table 2. Comparison of Rehabilitation, Teaching, and Treatment Approaches

	Rehabilitation	Teaching	Treatment
Focus	Daily living	Information, knowledge, and skills	Feelings and relationships
Assumptions	Psychosocial theory; client is the consumer; and client is disadvantaged	Cognitive/learning theory; parent is the consumer and client will conform	Personality and behavior theory; the professional is the provider; and the client is deviant
Goals	Restore and generate practical living skills; and modify consequences of impairment	Foster academic and preparatory skills; and remediate deficiencies	Reduce symptoms and conflicts; modify causes of disorder; and foster development
Assessment	Functional: work world; community living; self-care; self-advocacy; and adapting environments	Academic/social: norm reference; school world; and nonfamily world	Pathology: personal world; family world; and self adaptation

ment of children frequently omits a focus on future development. Rehabilitation considers disabled adults without a childhood past and tends to primarily focus on vocational goals.

APPLICATION OF THE REHABILITATION APPROACH TO PATIENTS

The usefulness of a rehabilitation approach with emotional disturbance is clearer when the prolonged use of traditional services has failed and chronicity has developed. Applying the proposed rehabilitation model, the treatment histories of two of the seven adolescents described at the beginning of the chapter are presented.

Case of Rondy

Rondy was a 17-year-old girl whose past and present mental status and adjustment were being reviewed by the Department of Mental Health to justify financial support of long-term residential placement. This request for placement had been made by her parents on the recommendation of her psychiatrist.

Rondy was interviewed by a psychiatrist together with a social work evaluator of the Department of Mental Health. Rondy was uncomfortable talking about herself and her feelings throughout the interview. She acknowledged having felt depressed for a long time and reluctantly admitted having made two suicidal attempts with pills, which led to two psychiatric hospitalizations. Presently, she is taking antidepressant medication. Following hospitalization a year ago, Rondy had been seeing a woman psychiatrist whom she liked. However, Rondy seemed to have little insight into her problems. She said she hated school where she had experienced failure for 10 years. She had received special education services since the first grade. Currently, she preferred to stay home and miss school. Her friends tended to be low achievers and involved in drug and alcohol use. She worked in a clothing store 15 hours a week, on Saturday and Sunday. Sometimes work would become confusing because she had difficulty understanding what she was supposed to do. Her thoughts about the future were ill defined and vague. She was physiologically mature and attractively dressed and groomed. She was sexually active without using birth control measures. No pregnancies had resulted to date.

Rondy was one of three adopted children, having older and younger brothers. Her father had a progressive degenerative hip disability that had limited his ability to work. Her mother was the main wage earner of the family. In general the children were viewed by their parents as not having lived up to parental expectations.

In reviewing Rondy's clinical records, one was impressed by the repeated diagnostic studies at various university tertiary-care facilities. Remedial education and treatment efforts had been numerous, but little attention had been paid to strength and skill development. There had been little preparatory training for the adult world of work, independent living, community involvement, and pragmatic literacy and computational skills. Therapeutic and educational assistance had remained primarily focused on her impairments.

In summary, Rondy appeared to have a learning disability associated with borderline intelligence and minimal brain damage. She was chronically depressed, angry, and frustrated, in part based on repeated ongoing failure experiences. Her family appeared to be dysfunctional, whereas she was related to a peer group that supported marginal adjustment and substance misuse. Her work experiences were fraught with difficulties as well. What was now being professionally recommended was treatment and remediation in a segregated, restrictive child-oriented setting with individual psychotherapy, special education, and supportive milieu. Little attention was directed toward adult occupation and living skills and was therefore likely to maintain frustration, failure, and depression.

Case of William

William was a 15½-year-old adolescent who had been recently discharged from a psychiatric hospitalization of 16 weeks duration. He was in limbo at home awaiting a residential placement to materialize without the development of a transitional program. Psychiatric consultation was requested to assess the adequacy of antidepressant medication prescribed during his hospitalization.

William was seen with a social worker. He presented an unusual appearance with delayed pubescence. He was smoking cigarettes from a pack given to him, reportedly by a teacher at school. He was attending a special education class (resource room) 2 hours a day in the morning and from 10:30 A.M. and had no scheduled activities. He denied having any current difficulties but refused to talk about the recent past. He did not respond to inquiries about future plans. Although he tested reality adequately, it was not possible to develop a trusting alliance with him during the interview.

His mother joined the interview and felt overwhelmed about the management and control of his behaviors. For years, William had been periodically expelled or suspended by school for surly and uncooperative behavior and fighting. He was frequently picked up by the police for stealing and for running away. Currently, from 11:00 A.M. on each day, mother had to monitor and control his behaviors. William spent much time in his room listening to loud rock music and watching TV. He took occasional trips to the store.

The initial psychiatric impression was that William had a borderline personality disorder with periodic episodes of psychotic behavior. Antipsychotic medication was therefore prescribed in addition to an antidepressant. An extended structured day of school and other activities were also advised, but it was difficult to enlist the cooperation of other community agencies in William's transitional placement at home.

Two weeks later, William was seen again in emergency psychiatric consultation because of an episode of firesetting and bizarre disorganized behaviors. His mother and her boyfriend were frightened and unable to control him. Mental status evaluation affirmed psychotic thinking and irrational behaviors with a depressed mood and paranoid ideation. William was committed for hospitalization with maternal agreement.

In reviewing his records, an extensive report from the recent 16-week hospitalization showed the severity of William's disturbance based on his difficulties in adjusting to both dormitory and classroom life, on behavioral observations, on neurological assessments, and on extensive psychodiagnostic testing. Long-term residential treatment was recommended for "massive interventions to cope with emotional, physical, and intellectual deficits" even though William had responded poorly to these same hospital interventions. Although the need for prevocational and life skills training was recognized, it was not incorporated in short- and long-term treatment recommendations.

Past history indicated that when William was 11 years old, his parents were divorced after a stormy marriage. His father had no contact with the family following the divorce. A review of his clinical records showed that developmental and behavior difficulties had been noted and evaluated periodically since infancy. William was enrolled in special education and mental health programs as early as first grade for learning difficulties and behavior problems at school and home. Over the years, his behaviors had become progressively more extreme including truancy, running away, stealing, drug and alcohol use, firesetting, physical abuse of siblings, and verbal abuse of adults. Medications and different psychological treatments had been attempted for a long time without much success.

In summary, William was an adolescent with a severe psychiatric disorder of long standing. He had normal intelligence but had learning difficulties associated with mild neurological impairment. Over his childhood and adolescent years, more restrictive school placements were made, supported by repeated and extensive psychodiagnostic studies in a number of urban university hospital facilities. William's hospitalization was the culmination of many years of failure and frustration to modify deviant and maladaptive behaviors.

Rehabilitation Perspectives

Both 17-year-old Rondy and 15-year-old William needed a greater emphasis in their program on (a) functional academics; (b) vocational assessment, planning, and experience—for Rondy, an assessment of why she found work confusing and how to improve her performance, and for William, a basic plan for matching his skills to a potential work environment; (c) appropriate psychoactive medication to help them function more adequately in nonresidential environments; (d) the facilitation and pursuit of recreational and leisure time activities; (e) cognitive social skills training; and (f) assistance to their parents in the management of extreme behaviors. These suggested program revisions might not have produced changes in the personality structures of Rondy and William; in fact such changes would not be the intent of the interventions. Interventions guided by a developmental rehabilitation approach would focus on helping such children and adolescents cope more adequately with the practicalities of everyday life in a developmental perspective.

SUMMARY

In this chapter, a number of clinical examples along with research evidence indicate that seriously emotionally disturbed children are underserved and at times poorly and ineffectively served. Part of that state of affairs may stem from omissions within the traditional services of special education and mental health. Particularly neglected is the concept of transitions and transitional services at times of role and setting changes. Also neglected is a life-span developmental orientation.

A developmental rehabilitation model is proposed that integrates contributions from rehabilitation and child and adult development. This model is based on a number of propositions:

1. Seriously emotionally disturbed children have impairments that in many instances cannot be cured and remediated.
2. The consequences of impairment to the person that is disability and the consequences of the disability with the environment that is the handicap can be assessed and altered through rehabilitation interventions that are not commonly used.
3. Such services will be most effective if they are interdisciplinary and involve coordinated service delivery networks.

These proposed ideas challenge traditional methods of service and training that have received a high degree of acceptance and economic success without proven effectiveness.

REFERENCES

American Academy of Child Psychiatry. (1983). *Child psychiatry: A plan for the coming decades.* Washington, DC: American Academy of Child Psychiatry.

American Psychiatric Association. (1981). *Statistical manual of mental disorders* (2nd ed. rev.). Washington, DC: American Psychiatric Association.

Anthony, W. A., Cohen, M., & Cohen, B. (1983). Philosophy, treatment process, and principles of the psychiatric rehabilitation approach. In L. Bachrach (Ed.), *New directions for mental health services: Deinstitutionalization, 17,* 67–79. San Francisco: Jossey-Bass.

Baenen, R. S., Stephens, M. A. P., & Glenwick, D. S. (1986). Outcome in psychoeducational day school programs: A review. *American Journal of Orthopsychiatry, 56,* 263–270.

Blom, G. E., Farley, G. K., & Ekanger, C. (1973). A psychoeducational treatment program: Its characteristics and results. In G. E. Blom and G. K. Farley (Eds.), *Report on activities of the Day Care Center of the University of Colorado Medical Center to the Commonwealth Foundation* (pp. 65–81), Denver: University of Colorado Medical Center Press.

Blom, G. E. (1982). *The impact of the disabled child on the family.* Lecture series to parents and special educators of the Ingham Intermediate School District, Mason, Michigan.

Blom, S. D., Lininger, R. S., & Charlesworth, W. R. (1987). Ecological observations of emotionally and behaviorally disordered students: A new method. *American Journal of Orthopsychiatry, 57,* 49–59.

Blotcky, M. J., Dimperio, T. L., & Gossett, J. T. (1984). Follow-up of children treated in psychiatric hospitals: A review of studies. *American Journal of Psychiatry, 141,* 1499–1507.

Brady, J. P. (1984a). Social skills training for psychiatric patients: I. Concepts, methods, and clinical results. *American Journal of Psychiatry, 141,* 333–340.

Brady, J. P. (1984b). Social skills training for psychiatric patients: II. Clinical outcome studies. *American Journal of Psychiatry, 141,* 491–498.

Bronfenbrenner, U. (1979). *The ecology of human development: Experiments by nature and design.* Cambridge: Harvard University Press.

Chiba, C. (1984). Children's attitudes towards emotionally disturbed peers. In R. L. Jones (Ed.), *Attitudes and attitude change in special education: Theory and practice.* (pp. 171–183), Reston, VA.: CEC Monograph.

Edgar, E. (1985). How do special education students fare after they leave school. *Exceptional Children, 511,* 470–473.

Federal Register. (1984). Cooperative models for planning and developing transitional services, 84.158C.

Gabel, S., & Finn, M. (1986). Outcome of children's day-treatment programs: Review of the literature and recommendations for future research. *International Journal of Partial Hospitalization, 3,* 261–271.

Gillespie, E. B., and Turnbull, A. P. (1983). It's my IEP—involving students in the planning process. *Teaching Exceptional Children, 16,* 27–29.

Goffman, E. (1963). *Stigma: Notes on the management of spoiled identity.* Englewood Cliffs, NJ: Prentice-Hall.

Gossett, J. T., Lewis, J. M., & Barnhart, F. D. (1983). *To find a way: The outcome of hospital treatment of disturbed adolescents.* New York: Brunner/Mazel.

Gould, M. S., Wunsch-Hitzig, R., & Dohrenwend, B. (1981). Estimating the prevalence of childhood psychopathology. *Journal of the American Academy of Child Psychiatry, 20,* 462–476.

Gracula, V., Rosenthal, R. H., Curtiss, G., & Marohn, R. C. (1984). Dropout from adolescent psychotherapy. *Journal of the American Academy of Child Psychiatry, 23,* 562–568.

Halpern, A. S. (1985). Transition: A look at the foundations. *Exceptional Children, 51,* 479–486.

Hasazi, S. B., Gordon, L. R., & Roe, C. A. (1985). Factors associated with the employment status of handicapped youth exiting high school from 1979 to 1983. *Exceptional Children, 51,* 455–469.

Hobbs, N. (1982). *The troubled and troubling child: Re-education and mental health education and human service programs for children and youth.* San Francisco: Jossey-Bass.

Hobbs, N., Egerton, J., & Matheny, M. H. (1975). Classifying children. *Children Today, 4*(4), 21–25.

Joint Commission of Mental Health of Children. (1969). *Crisis in child mental health: Challenge for the 1970's.* New York: Harper & Row.

Knitzer, J., & Olson, L. (1982). *Unclaimed children.* Washington, DC: Children's Defense Fund.

Lewis, D. O., Shanok, S. S., Klatskin, E., & Osborne, J. R. (1980). The undoing of residential treatment. *Journal of the American Academy of Child Psychiatry, 19,* 160–171.

Lotto, L. S. (1985). The unfinished agenda: Report from the National Commission on Secondary-Vocational Education. *Phi Delta Kappan, 66,* 563–573.

Lourie, L. S., & Katz-Leavy, J. (1987). Severely emotionally disturbed children and adolescents. In W. Menninger & G. Hanna (Eds.), *The chronic mental patient/II* (pp. 159–185). Washington, DC: American Psychiatric Press.

Maddox, M., Edgar, E., & Levine, P. (1984). *Post school status of graduates of special education.* Working paper, Experimental Education Unit, University of Washington, Seattle.

Mithaug, D. E., Horiuchi, C. N., & Fanning, P. N. (1985). A report on the Colorado statewide follow up survey of special education students. *Exceptional Children, 51,*(5), 397–404.

National Association of State Directors of Special Education (1985). *SED findings (Contract No. 300-83-0134 and 300-82-001).* Washington, DC: U.S. Department of Education.

Pfeiffer, S. (Ed.). (1984). *Clinical child psychology: An introduction to theory, research and practice.* New York: Grune & Stratton.

Prentice-Dunn, S., Wilson, D. R., & Lyman, R. D. (1981). Client factors related to outcome in a residential and day treatment program for children. *Journal of Clinical Child Psychology, 10,* 188–191.

Rehab Brief. (1983). People with chronic schizophrenia: Their rehabilitation outlook. Vol. VI, No. 2, February.

Rutter, M. (1983). Psychological therapies in child psychiatry: Issues and prospects. *Psychological Medicine, 12,* 723–740.

Safilios-Rothschild, C. (1970). *The sociology and social psychology of disability and rehabilitation.* New York: Random House.

Shaffer, D. (1984). Notes on psychotherapy research among children and adolescents. *Journal of the American Academy of Child Psychiatry, 23,* 552–561.

Tringo, J. L. (1972). The hierarchy of preference toward desirability groups. *Journal of Special Education, 1,* 295–306.

Wehman, P., Kregel, J., & Barcus, J. M. (1985). From school to work: A vocational transitional model for handicapped students. *Exceptional Children, 52,* 25–37.

Will, M. C. (1984a). Let us pause and reflect—but not too long. *Exceptional Children, 51,* 11–16.

Will, M. C. (1984b). Bridges from school to working life. Programs for the handicapped. *Clearinghouse on the Handicapped,* March/April, 1–5.

World Health Organization. (1980). *International classification of impairments, disabilities and handicaps.* Geneva.

Wright, B. A. (1983). *Physical disability: A psychological approach* (2nd ed.). New York: Harper & Row.

Zimet, S. G., & Farley, G. K. (1985). Day treatment for children in the United States. *Journal of the American Academy of Child Psychiatry, 24,* 732–738.

Zimet, S. G., Farley, G. K., Silver, J., Hebert, F. B., Robb, E. D., Ekanger, C., & Smith, D. (1980). Behavior and personality changes in emotionally disturbed children in a psychoeducational day treatment center. *Journal of the American Academy of Child Psychiatry, 19,* 240–256.

5

Child and Adolescent Day Treatment

A General Systems Theory Perspective

LAUREL J. KISER and DAVID B. PRUITT

A general systems theory perspective (von Bertalanffy, 1968; Hoffman, 1981; Miller, 1965) is entirely compatible with day treatment that consists of multiple components or subsystems. "A system is usually thought of as a whole consisting of interdependent and interacting parts or a set of units with relationships among them" (Compton & Gallaway, 1979). Day treatment is a system with component parts as well as being a subsystem in the larger mental-health-care organization. An appreciation of the principles of systems theory, including the importance of reciprocity and interaction among members, is essential to the optimal functioning of a day treatment program. Biological, social, psychological, individual, educational, family, small-group, program milieu, organizational, and community issues must be attended to and recognized. According to Isenberg (1983), such a multisystem approach is required for effective day treatment. It is believed that trying to isolate and treat a single malfunctioning subsystem is likely to be either incorrect or at the very least, inadequate.

In September 1982, a pilot free-standing day treatment program was opened at the University of Tennessee Center for the Health

LAUREL J. KISER and DAVID B. PRUITT • Day Treatment Program, University of Tennessee, Memphis, Tennessee 38105.

Sciences. Seed money was provided by the university, with a clear understanding that this was an interest-free loan. The initial mandate of the day treatment program was simply to become a financially self-sufficient program as quickly as possible. A total of 16 patients, 8 children and 8 adolescents with moderate to severe psychopathology, were accepted into the program. The program was based on a general systems approach and will be described in the following section.

ORGANIZATIONAL SUBSYSTEM

Staffing Patterns

From an organizational standpoint, it is essential that the staff consist of a multidisciplinary team to maintain a systems perspective. Disciplines usually represented on the team include psychiatry, psychology, social work, education, recreation, and nursing. The staffing patterns within the team are likely to vary from program to program in terms of professional makeup and role functions, however. The workings of the multidisciplinary treatment team can be compared to the structure within a healthy and productive family system. Functioning of the multidisciplinary team is believed to be an important factor that contributes to the effectiveness of the overall system. Dysfunctional interactional patterns and unresolved conflict among staff can reverberate throughout the therapeutic system. Differentiation of roles is a necessity to assure healthy functioning (Pugh, 1982). Each staff member functions in a role that has specific responsibilities associated with it. Examples include differentiation of roles and responsibilities between clinical and direct care staff as well as differentiation of therapeutic roles, that is, individual versus family therapist. Each member of the professional family requires a distinctive job description. These job descriptions are developed as a joint effort between the administrative supervisor and a staff member.

Organizational Structure

Also, when any group of professionals works together as a team, a clear power hierarchy has to be established. The dynamics characterizing this power structure and the hierarchy creating these dynamics are worthy of discussion. In our program, the power structure is organized on three levels. Level 1, the administration and clinical management of the program is handled by the program director (psychologist/administrator) and the medical director (child psychiatrist). They are co-equals, each with clearly defined responsibilities for different and respective aspects of the program. The second level of authority in the organizational hierarchy is the program coordinator (floor coordinator) whose responsibilities within the power hierarchy include scheduling activities and assuring patient treatment. This person therefore provides a liaison between administration and direct care personnel. The third level of authority in the organizational hierarchy is comprised of the direct patient care personnel. We have found this three-tiered organizational structure to be highly effective and speculate that its efficacy depends upon regular team meetings, staff development, and individual supervision. These practices appear not only to enhance interrelations but provide one key solution to the problem of staff burnout. Staff burnout is reduced due to the healthy functioning of the team and good relationships that develop among the staff. Clear lines of communication are easily established that aid informal and formal means of providing input and support into difficult cases.

COMMUNITY SUBSYSTEM

Community commitment is a major component of a system-based day treatment program. The medical community cannot bear the sole responsibility for maintaining programs such as day treatment. Support for treatment must be broadly based and include other sources, for example, from community leaders, agencies, and businesses.

Advisory Board

We have found that development of a day treatment advisory board composed of prominent community members has provided a vital link with the community that has helped to assure the success of our program. Members of the board have included bankers, attorneys, local newscasters, public relations consultants, philanthropists, and educators. As its name indicates, its role is only advisory.

Sounding Board. These members provide a broader perspective than the day treatment administrators are likely to have developed and serve as a sounding board for new ideas and complicated policy issues. In their personal and professional contacts, they are in a position to foster good community relations, to establish program sponsors, and to negotiate cooperative relationships with other agencies.

Marketing Strategies. Public service announcements, magazine and newspaper articles, slide and video presentations, along with public relations receptions, have been initiated by our active community board. This helps in educating the community about day treatment as well as generating referrals. Another potential function of the board is providing resources for the program. As mentioned earlier, our program has a practical and philosophical mandate to be financially self-supporting. The community board can, if needed, help subsidize a program by development of a volunteer work force, by program equipment donations, and fund raising for scholarship positions. Also, board members who possess expertise in business and finance are helpful in the areas of budget, billing, and patient accounts.

Liaison with Community Agencies

Liaison with a variety of community agencies is essential for the support of day treatment. One means of support is the referral of patients. A comprehensive initial intake procedure, communication during the treatment process, and the fulfilled promise that all patients will be returned upon discharge to their original referral source are important factors in maintaining good relationships with the referring agency or individual. Community agencies such as the public and private schools, the Department of Human Services, the community mental health centers, the juvenile court, and the inpatient units, and the like are crucial support agencies in the development of a strong referral network. Close communication and negotiations with all these agencies help assure the day treatment program its place in the mainstream of the child and adolescent health and educational care delivery system.

Another critical function performed by the community subsystem is the formal establishment of close relationships with public and private school systems. Support from these school systems in providing transportation for some patients, teachers' salaries, accreditation, along with schoolbooks and supplies is essential.

Emergency Treatment

The community subsystem provides 24-hour emergency treatment for day treatment patients. Fulfillment of this function requires a good liaison among the pediatric hospitals and the psychiatric inpatient units for children and adolescents. The acknowledgment that some children and adolescents may need hospitalization and also that the day treatment staff will be available by beeper contact 24 hours a day/7 days a week helps reassure referral sources as well as parents that children at risk will receive appropriate care and supervision.

Third-Party Payers

The final dimension incorporated within the community subsystem involves the third-party payers such as private insurance companies and the governmental insurance sources like Medicaid. Negotiations with insurance companies and agencies such as Medicaid are mandatory for the establishment of a self-sufficient, self-supporting organization and essential for the future of day treatment services for children and adolescents. The main objective of negotiations is to introduce insurance companies to the concept of day treatment and to educate them about the population to be served as well as about the potential benefits of this type of treatment. The goal of such meetings is to enlist support for child and adolescent day treatment programs by convincing these funding agencies of the possibility as well as the desirability of lower health care costs and to establish criteria for admission and operation.

MILIEU SUBSYSTEM

The total program milieu, one subsystem often ignored in the therapeutic system, is critical to consider in the total system. Ecological psychology (Barker, 1968) presents one of the most cogent theories for studying complex behavior–environment interactions. According to this theory, a therapeutic milieu is a collection of settings in which behavior can take place. Each setting involves a certain space with its props, including furniture, books, games, along with a specific time span, a defined population, and patterns of behavior appropriate to that setting. According to ecological theory, behavior and the context or matrix of that behavior are inseparable. The characteristics of the setting are often thought to have a more powerful influence on the behavior of the individual than personality or intrapsychic dynamics. Thus, the structure and limits of an activity and the grouping of patients, staff, and environment must be carefully arranged in order to be therapeutic.

Utilizing Barker's theory, to structure the therapeutic milieu in day treatment involves considering each component of the program or segment of the child's day as comprising a separate behavior setting. For instance, joining the children for the morning community meeting creates a behavior setting different from the school activity time. It is important to identify each treatment component in order to adequately analyze or understand the patient's behavior. Finally, the nature of transition must be carefully engineered. For example, the transition for back-to-back activities with vastly different expectations, such as the transition from free time to group therapy, can become problematic. Thus the program must develop a sequence of settings that both provide the safety and security needed by the child and simultaneously stimulate the patient to grow and change.

Behavioral Program

In order to introduce the patient to appropriate patterns of behavior in general, as well as to establish an individualized program to satisfy each patient's needs, a behavioral program is utilized. Policies and rules are clearly outlined in a written manual for each child and adolescent. Additionally, each patient is challenged to accomplish a list of personal goals each day. Performance compliance with rules and expectations is monitored by a traditional behavioral-level system for the adolescent patients (Homme & Tosti, 1973) and a token system for the child patient (Ayllon & Azrin, 1968). This behavioral component of day treatment augments the psychotherapies by allowing a focus by the patient on both behavior and emotion.

Activities Therapy

Activities therapies, including recreation, art, movement, music, drama, and occupational therapy, are part of therapeutic milieu. In addition to these traditional therapies, social skills exercises and field trips are included. The goals for the activities therapy involve providing staff and peer support for appropriate behavior, experiencing success in areas other than academics, learning constructive uses of leisure time, and creating an environment that fosters social success by encouraging team work, cooperation, and persistence in completion of tasks. Free time, the most unstructured period of the day, is another part of activities therapy. It is often the most difficult time for staff to provide adequate supervision but is valuable for patients in terms of offering freedom of choice.

EDUCATIONAL SUBSYSTEM

Educational therapy is provided as a part of the program 3 to 4 hours each day as an opportunity for children to work toward a variety of goals, both academic and behavioral. This is the most highly structured setting during the entire day for the children and adolescents and hence may present extra challenges. The first educational priority of the staff at the time of admission is to assess current levels of basic academic functioning by use of standardized tests and other objective measures of academic performance. Then an individualized educational plan along with long- and short-term goals is developed for each child. The educational plan is designed to structure learning activities to meet individual needs, to stress adaptive learning skills, to remediate learning difficulties, and to foster success potential. Additionally, the educational component of day treatment aids children in dealing with common frustrations encountered in school settings. Appropriate school placement and follow-up upon discharge are final steps of the educational process.

FAMILY SUBSYSTEM

Another therapeutic subsystem to be dealt with in day treatment is the family subsystem. Family therapy in our program reflects a structural–strategic point of view (Haley, 1987; Minuchin, 1974; Stanton, 1981), with the major emphasis upon modification of the dysfunctional family structure so that the present symptoms exhibited by the child or adolescent will no longer need to be maintained. Establishing consistent rules and limits to be observed by the child, both at home and at the treatment center, is another goal of family work. Often meeting this objective involves contracting and extending consequences and reinforcements of appropriate behavior, for example, a level system, (Homme & Tosti, 1973) at home. In effect, parents are viewed as the co-therapists, the night shift, and therefore parent education and instruction in behavior management techniques are essential. A minimum of 1 hour per week of family therapy is recommended.

GROUP SUBSYSTEM

Group therapy should be provided for the children 1 to 2 hours daily. We do this at our center. Group therapy stimulates work on group dynamic issues involving cohesion, roles, norms, values, and so on. Generally, group therapy helps children develop problem solving and coping abilities through appropriate expression of feelings and experiences in a safe environment with adults and peers. Group work with adolescents involves sharing of problems and feelings, discussing and practicing alternatives, and actively negotiating conflict among peers and group leaders. The latency-age group work is a combination of talk therapy coupled with structured, interpreted play activities. Trust is built within groups by stressing the confidentiality of group matters to all members.

Children and adolescents participate on a weekly basis in another group session called peer and staff feedback. The group is run as a nonconfrontational feedback and evaluation forum. Each patient receives feedback from several peers and from any staff member. There is no discussion of the feedback allowed, although the patient is asked to evaluate his/her progress, behavior, work toward goals, level achieved, and so on. This setting provides an opportunity for the patient to integrate the various therapy subsystems in which he or she is working and provides an overall assessment of his or her functioning.

INDIVIDUAL SUBSYSTEM

Each child receives individual therapy 2 to 3 hours per week. The individual's work provides an opportunity for the patient to develop a close relationship with an adult other than a parent. The goal of this relationship is to facilitate the patient in working intensively on intrapsychic problem areas (Adams, 1982). Individual dynamics and conflicts are the major focus of this psychotherapy with an insight-oriented approach utilized for the adolescent population and more structured approaches, such as play therapy, used with the younger age groups. Content and process of individual therapy sessions are confidential unless the child or adolescent is a danger to self or to others. This assurance of confidentiality maintains appropriate boundaries around subsystems.

BIOLOGIC SUBSYSTEM

Because some disturbed children and adolescents are in need of psychoactive medication and/or general medical management, it is essential for any day treatment program to have a strong "biologic" (i.e., medical) component, ideally a child psychiatrist along with the various pediatric and other medical consultants. The child psychiatrist's responsibilities include those typically discharged by a physician on a psychiatric inpatient unit. These include a comprehensive psychiatric evaluation and detailed medical history as part of the standard admission workup. A diagnostic impression and a treatment plan are developed by the physician. The child psychiatrist serves as the integrator of the biopsychosocial aspects of the treatment program. Because of his or her medical expertise, he or she must be certain to address the biologic and physical aspect of the psychiatric illness (i.e., stomach aches as they relate to anxiety) as well as managing and triaging the patient's nonpsychiatric medical illnesses. The physician is involved in helping to provide appropriate discharge planning.

On nonpsychiatric medical hospital services, the physician typically makes daily "rounds" in order to monitor each patient's medical status. In a day treatment program, modification of these traditional rounds is the rule. Instead of interviewing every child each day to review psychiatric status, the child psychiatrist may more intensively meet with the child twice a week. Although the child psychiatrist may not see every child each day, he or she will indirectly monitor the daily medical care of each child through the direct care staff and the patient's primary psychotherapist. These nontraditional medical management rounds are essential in a day treatment program providing intensive psychiatric services to children and adolescents.

However, the physician's responsibility is not limited to the treatment of the individual patient's biologic functioning. Engel's (1977, 1980) biopsychosocial model is particularly consistent with a systems view of day treatment. For instance, in our program, the medical director, although responsible for the medical and clinical management of each patient, also serves as part of the total interdisciplinary team. He is involved in each component of the program, from staffing, community meetings, and supervision of clinical staff to individual, group, and family psychotherapies. This comprehensive involvement allows the child psychiatrist to be a true practitioner of the biopsychosocial model. In addition to providing treatment, a strong medical component in the day treatment program is essential for other more practical reasons such as accreditation of the program. Some states require structured psychiatric services such as a day treatment program to be licensed. This licensure requires the presence of varying degrees of medical psychiatric input. Development of future accreditation mechanisms by such national organizations as the Joint Commission on Accreditation of Health Care Organizations (JCAHO) requires a strong medical presence. Reimbursement by third party payers is often dependent upon medical personnel, procedures, diagnoses, and overall effective medical treatment.

INTEGRATING SUBSYSTEMS

Systems thinking necessitates using a multidisciplinary team and a variety of therapeutic modalities to treat moderately to severely disturbed children and adolescents in day treatment. Use of this approach raises several therapeutic issues that cannot be ignored. One is the issue of confidentiality among therapeutic modalities, and another is the involvement of multiple therapists with any patient. Although related, the two create separate concerns for consideration.

When working with a team approach, there is always the question of who shares what information with whom. One basic tenant of systems theory specifies that no subsystem can be treated in isolation. Accordingly, a certain amount of information must be shared in order for the various components of treatment to be well integrated and meaningfully related. The doctrine of confidentiality usually dictates that information shared between therapist and patient remains private. What are the limits of confidentiality within a team from a systems perspective? We have generated several rules to aid therapists in determining what can and should be shared:

1. The treatment of any child/adolescent and family is held strictly confidential by the program as a whole.
2. Each patient and family is informed that a team approach is used and information about their case is shared. Patients and families who have difficulties with this model are encouraged to discuss these concerns with each of their therapists and express specific reservations about information to be shared.
3. The amount of information shared is often determined on an individual, case-by-case basis. For instance, an adolescent admitted with paranoid symptomatology may require an individual therapist who maintains strict confidentiality while a trusting relationship is built; whereas a manipulative, acting-out adolescent may necessitate a great deal of open communication among staff members in order for appropriate limits to be maintained.

4. Confidentiality within the patient community is stressed, especially in group psychotherapy settings. Patients are encouraged to respect the privacy of fellow group members by not discussing group issues outside of the group setting.
5. In situations where issues and information need to be shared between therapeutic modalities, for example between individual and family psychotherapy, the patient is urged to initiate discussion of these topics with therapists providing appropriate support and guidance.

Involvement of more than one therapist with the same patient (such as a different group therapist, individual therapist, and family therapist) has both advantages and disadvantages from a systems perspective. The use of one versus multiple therapists is a decision that is best made based upon individual case dynamics. For example, with latency-age children, it may be therapeutic for the individual and family therapist to be the same person, whereas for an adolescent trying to differentiate from family, two separate therapists may be indicated.

When multiple therapists are involved with the same patient, it is important to evaluate how those therapists integrate into the family system. Communication between therapists is essential in order to prevent splitting of the therapeutic team, a great hazard when dealing with dysfunctional families. Additionally, it is crucial that the therapists maintain role boundaries and encourage family members to utilize each therapeutic modality appropriately.

CONCLUSION

General systems theory provides a good theoretical background for a child/adolescent day treatment program. The theory states that many different areas of a person's life (i.e., family, peers, school, work, neighbors, church) influence one's functioning. Having adopted this perspective, day treatment provides a setting to treat every aspect of the child or adolescent system while maintaining a therapeutic environment throughout each day.

General systems theory introduces complexity to the therapeutic treatment process by broadening the range of possibilities and focus. Because of the emphasis on multiple systems interventions, there is a constant challenge to adequately diagnose and assess problems from a multilevel perspective. The traditional individual diagnosis has validity only if the individual system is the underlying major dysfunction. General systems theory demands appraisal of a variety of systems, not only the biological or individual variables, but also the family, group, milieu, educational, community, and organizational variables. Finally, the theory itself sharpens awareness of such fundamental ethical questions as *what* one is to change, what *can* be changed, what one has a *right* to change, and *who* is responsible for creating the opportunity for change.

REFERENCES

Adams, P. L. (1982). *A primer of child psychotherapy* (2nd ed.). Boston: Little, Brown.

Ayllon, T., & Azrin, N. H. (1968). *The token economy: A motivational system for therapy and rehabilitation.* New York: Appleton-Century-Crofts.

Barker, R. G. (1968). *Ecological psychology.* Stanford: Stanford University Press.

Bertalanffy, L. von (1968). *General system theory: Foundations, development, applications.* New York: George Braziller.

Compton, B., & Gallaway, B. (1979). *Social work processes.* Homewood: Dorsey Press.

Engel, G. L. (1977). The need for a new medical model: A challenge for biomedicine. *Science, 196,* 129–136.

Engel, G. L. (1980). The clinical application of the biopsychosocial model. *American Journal of Psychiatry, 137,* 535–544.

Haley, J. (1987). *Problem-solving therapy* (2nd ed.). San Francisco: Jossey-Bass.

Hoffman, L. (1981). *Foundations of family therapy.* New York: Basic Books.

Homme, L., & Tosti, D. (1973). *Behavior technology: Motivation and contingency management.* San Rafael, CA: Individual Learning Systems.

Isenberg, D. P. (1983). A systematic-developmental model of day treatment for young adult chronic patients. *International Journal of Partial Hospitalization, 2,* 113–124.

Miller, J. G. (1965). Living systems: Basic concepts. *Behavioral Science, 10,* 193–237.

Minuchin, S. (1974). *Families and family therapy.* Cambridge, MA: Harvard University Press.

Pugh, R. L. (1982). Resolving boundary problems among therapists. *International Journal of Family Therapy, 4*(1), 31–39.

Stanton, M. D. (1981). An integrated structural-strategic approach to family therapy. *Journal of Marital and Family Therapy, 7,* 427–439.

6

A Behavioral Model of Day Treatment

ROBERT D. LYMAN and STEVEN PRENTICE-DUNN

INTRODUCTION

Day treatment programs for children with psychiatric disorders have been identified by Zimet and Farley (1985) as being based on several theoretical models, including those with primarily psychodynamic, developmental therapy, and behavioral orientations. This chapter focuses on a program based primarily on a behavioral model. The rationale for this model will be presented, and the use of both individual behavioral interventions and comprehensive contingency management systems will be discussed. The specific contingency management systems utilized at Brewer-Porch Children's Center will be described in detail.

The Rationale for the Behavioral Model

A theoretical model that appears ideally suited for utilization in children's psychiatric day treatment is behaviorism. Behavior therapy has been shown to be effective in dealing with a wide range of childhood psychiatric disturbances, ranging from self-mutilative and psychotic symptoms (Allen & Harris, 1966) to phobic reactions (Tahmisian & McReynolds, 1971) and conduct disorders (Madsen & Madsen,

ROBERT D. LYMAN and STEVEN PRENTICE-DUNN • Department of Psychology, University of Alabama, Tuscaloosa, Alabama 35487.

1972). A major limitation of outpatient behavior therapy, however, is the amount of therapeutic conditioning that can take place in a therapy session compared to the amount of nontherapeutic conditioning that occurs in the child's natural environment. Outpatient behavior therapists have often had to rely on parents and teachers to implement behavior therapy procedures without supervision in an effort to expand their therapeutic impact. With day treatment, such procedures can be implemented by trained staff in a tightly controlled environment, with implementation responsibility only gradually shifted to less trained individuals in the child's natural environment. Similarly, initial behavioral assessment, which relies heavily on direct observation, can be accomplished by trained personnel rather than relying on the imprecise and sometimes subjective observations of parents, teachers, and others.

Day treatment also offers advantages over inpatient hospitalization for the behavior therapist. First, day treatment, by virtue of the fact that the child spends one-half to three-fourths of each day in his or her natural environment, is much more conducive to generalization of treatment effects than inpatient hospitalization. Second, problems in transfer of therapeutic conditioning can be detected earlier and remediated, rather than only being detected at the end of hospitalization when remediation may not be possible. Third, parents often feel excluded by their child's hospitalization and may be less willing to learn and implement behavior therapy techniques than if their child is seen daily in day treatment. Fourth, there are often differences in a child's perception of his/her role in inpatient treatment versus day treatment that may affect treatment outcome. Children in hospitals commonly feel more passive and less responsible for their treatment, whereas children in more "schoollike" surroundings, such as day treatment, are more invested in their own progress. These attitudinal differences can be critical in the success of a behavior therapy program. Finally, staff in inpatient programs are predominantly medically trained and may have little use for behavioral etiological explanations and treatment procedures, preferring the familiarity of the medical model, with its primarily organic etiological explanations and somatic treatments. By contrast, day treatment programs are often less philosophically committed to the medical model and usually have many more staff whose training and experience are in education and community mental health and who are more knowledgeable and comfortable regarding behavioral approaches to assessment and treatment.

BEHAVIORAL MODELS

There are basically two formats that could be described as behavioral day treatment. The first of these consists of a traditionally structured day treatment program within which isolated behavioral therapy procedures are implemented. Time during the day may be largely occupied with educational activities, ADL (activities of daily living) training, social skills training, verbal and activity therapies, and recreation. Within this context, individual children may be exposed to behavior therapy procedures.

BEHAVIORAL INTERVENTIONS

The literature is replete with reports of the effective use of behavioral interventions within school settings (Rickard, Willis, & Clements, 1974; Wielkiewicz, 1986). Many of these have been adopted for use in day treatment programs. The following provides a brief discussion of each type of intervention.

Aversive Conditioning

Contingent Electric Shock. Punishment has been used in a number of different ways to produce behavior change in children and adolescents with psychiatric disorders. Contingent electric shock has been used almost exclusively with psychotic, autistic, and mentally retarded children and usually only with severely maladaptive and/or dangerous behaviors. Usually less intrusive treatment procedures have been previously tried and have proven ineffective (Gelfand & Hartmann, 1975; Risley, 1968). Tate and Baroff (1966) employed a painful electric shock administered to the leg of a 9-year-old psychotic boy whenever he banged his head or punched himself in the face. At the same time, noninjurious behavior was rewarded with praise. After 167 days, the self-injurious behavior was completely eliminated. Lovaas and Simmons (1969) were similarly able to eliminate self-injurious behaviors in three severely retarded children through the use of contingent electric shock. Other problem behaviors that have been effectively dealt with through this procedure include tantrums (Lovaas, Frietag, Kinder, Rubenstein, Schaeffer, & Simmons, 1966), aggression (Brandsma & Stein, 1973) and eating paper (Hamilton & Standahl, 1969).

Noxious Stimuli. Another aversive conditioning procedure that has been reported in the literature is the use of noxious stimuli such as lemon juice, ammonia capsules, and noise. Sajwaj, Libet, and Agras (1974) reported that squirting concentrated lemon juice into the mouth of a 6-month-old infant when the child began rumination was successful in eliminating this potentially life-threatening behavior. Conway and Bucher (1974) found that squirting shaving cream into the mouth of a profoundly retarded child, contingent on the beginning of tantrum behavior, was effective in eliminating this behavior. Altman, Haavik, and Cook (1978) report that holding a broken ammonia capsule under a mentally retarded child's nose was an effective intervention when the child began hair pulling.

Verbal Reprimands. Several investigators (Baumeister & Forehand, 1972; O'Leary, Kaufman, Kass, & Drabman, 1970) have shown that verbal reprimands can serve as effective aversive stimuli in reducing inappropriate behaviors. However, Madsen, Becker, Thomas, Koser, and Plager (1968) found that the more first-grade teachers verbally reprimanded students for being out of their seats, the more the students were out of their seats. Obviously, caution is advised when using verbal reprimands as an aversive stimulus. In some cases, they may function to produce the opposite of the desired result due to the attention such procedures direct toward the child.

Overcorrection. This punishment procedure follows the demonstration of a maladaptive behavior with enforced restitution (cleanup, pickup, etc.) and repeated practice of a more adaptive response to the same situation. For example, should a child knock over a chair that is in his/her way, she or he might be required to set the chair back up and practice walking past it or gently moving it aside 10 to 30 times. Overcorrection has been used to eliminate inappropriate mouthing of objects for which an oral hygiene procedure constituted the restitution and positive practice components (Foxx & Azrin, 1973). Overcorrection also has been used to eliminate head-banging with arm and head exercises required following the maladaptive behavior (Harris & Romanczyk, 1976). Epstein, Doke, Sajwaj, Sorrell, and Rimmer (1974) demonstrated that overcorrection was an effective procedure even when the restitution and positive practice were not logically related to the maladaptive behavior.

Negative Practice. Related to overcorrection is the technique of negative practice, in which a child is required to repeat a maladaptive behavior with little or no rest until an aversive level of fatigue builds up. Thus the maladaptive behavior is punished with fatigue. Walton (1961) required a young boy with multiple tics to engage in prolonged practice of his primary tic. This intervention proved effective in eliminating the tics. With another child, Walton (1964) also used negative practice in conjunction with medication to reduce head shaking, hiccups, and explosive exhaling. The improvement was maintained at a 5-month follow-up. Clark (1966) treated two children with Tourette's syndrome with negative practice and found that it was highly effective in reducing the frequency of obscene utterances. However, Lahey, McNees, and McNees (1973) were unable to reduce a 10-year-old boy's obscene vocalizations through the use of negative practice. They then switched to a time-out program, which was effective in reducing the behavior. Negative practice is not commonly used with child behavioral problems, perhaps because of the practitioner's hesitation about having children practice (and presumably strengthen) maladaptive behavior patterns. More research is clearly needed to determine the usefulness of this technique.

Response Cost. Monetary or behavioral penalties for inappropriate behavior are called *response cost procedures.* Sanok and Streifel (1979), for instance, treated an electively mute 11-year-old girl by first presenting her with a number of pennies and then asking her questions. When she failed to respond, a penny was taken from her. This procedure, along with positive reinforcers for speech, was effective in getting the child to speak again.

Alexander, Corbett, and Smigel (1976) gave delinquent adolescents weekly lunch money and then withdrew it for the day from all subjects if anyone did not attend all of their classes. This procedure proved highly effective. Clark, Greene, Macrae, McNees, Davis, and Risley (1977) used 5-cent fines for disruptive behavior while shopping with children who had previously been told they would have 50 cents to spend at the end of shopping. Response cost, in the form of token fines, is frequently used as a component of a token economy (Doty, McInnis, & Paul, 1974). Kazdin (1973) compared the effectiveness of several procedures in reducing speech dysfluencies in mentally retarded adults. Among these were (a) a token fine procedure, (b) an aversive conditioning procedure (loud noise), (c) information feedback, and (d) a no-treatment control. The token fine procedure proved to be the most effective intervention.

In conclusion, the aversive conditioning techniques discussed are powerful tools that can produce significant behavioral change. However, it has often been cautioned (e.g., Gelfand & Hartmann, 1975) that such techniques should be utilized as a last resort when interventions based on positive reinforcement have not been successful. When aversive conditioning strategies are implemented, careful consideration must be given to the rights and welfare of the child involved.

Time-Out. Another effective behavioral intervention is time-out from positive reinforcement, in which inappropriate behaviors are followed by removal from peer attention and other positive reinforcers. Usually, this removal is effected by placement in a hallway, adjoining room, or specially constructed "time-out room" until appropriate behavior is demonstrated. Drabman and Spitalnik (1973) used an identical technique that they called "contingent social isolation" to reduce disruptive classroom behaviors in boys at a psychiatric hospital. Baseline data were gathered on three disruptive behaviors: inappropriate vocalizations, aggression, and being out of seat without permission. Out-of-seat and aggressive behaviors resulted in the child spending 10 minutes in a small bare room near the classroom, after which he or she was allowed to rejoin the class. Results indicated that out-of-seat behaviors decreased from 34% of the time during baseline to 11% of the time following the social isolation intervention. Aggression decreased from 2.8% of the time during baseline to only 0.37% of the time following intervention. Inappropriate vocalizations, which were not treated with social isolation, decreased only slightly, from 32% during baseline to 28% following the social isolation intervention with the other two behaviors. It is worth noting that when the social isolation contingency was removed, the occurrence rates of aggressive and out-of-seat behaviors increased only slightly. Time-out procedures are widely used in psychiatric treatment facilities for children (Wilson & Lyman, 1982) and can be implemented in a variety of ways.

Positive Conditioning

Positive Reinforcement. Positive reinforcement for appropriate behavior has been shown to be one of the most effective interventions with school behavior problems. Bijou and Baer (1963) found that adult attention contingent on social interaction increased the amount of time spent in conversation by a withdrawn 4-year-old from 10% to over 60%. Stone (1970) used a primary reinforcer, cookies, to reduce disruptive classroom behavior in seven boys with cerebral palsy. Cookies were offered for initial 5-minute intervals of appropriate behavior with the interval later lengthened to 15 minutes. After 2½ months, however, inappropriate behavior increased again. The boys had evidently became satiated on the cookies, and they had lost their reinforcement value. A different reinforcer was necessary to maintain behavioral improvement.

Activity reinforcers, or the opportunity to engage in preferred activities as a result of demonstrating appropriate behavior, have also been used effectively with children (Premack, 1965). Blinder, Freeman, and Stunkard (1970) found that making the opportunity to engage in physical activity (e.g., walking and exercise) contingent upon weight gain, resulted in rapid increases in weight for several adolescent females with anorexia nervosa. The weight gain had been maintained at an 8- to 10-month follow-up. Homme, DeBaca, Devine, Steinhorst, and Rickert (1963) allowed three disruptive children in a nursery school classroom to run and scream after they sat quietly for a period of time. Within a few days, the children were sitting quietly for substantially longer periods of time. Other preferred behaviors that have been effectively used as reinforcers for children include television watching, going to a store or sporting event, and interacting with peers and adults. Usually, a brief period of observation can quickly establish which are a child's preferred activities.

Behavioral Contracts. Positive reinforcers and the requirements for earning them can be explicitly stated in a contingency contract. Homme (1970) identified 10 basic rules for effective behavioral contracting:

Rule 1. The contract payoff (reward) should be immediate.
Rule 2. Initial contracts should call for and reward small approximations of the desired behavior.
Rule 3. Reward frequently with small amounts.
Rule 4. The contract should call for and reward accomplishments rather than obedience.
Rule 5. Reward the performance as it occurs.
Rule 6. The contract must be fair.
Rule 7. The terms of the contract must be clear.
Rule 8. The contract must be honest.
Rule 9. The contract must be positive.
Rule 10. Contracting as a method must be used systematically.

Stuart (1974) described the use of a behavioral contract with social privileges as a reinforcer to decrease delinquent behaviors in a 16-year-old girl. Dinoff, Serum, and Rickard (1974) used behavioral contracts to decrease disruptive and rebellious behaviors in three adolescent girls at a therapeutic summer camp, and Dinoff, Rickard, and Colwick (1974) used a series of behavioral contracts with activity reinforcers to effect weight loss (30 pounds over a 7-week period) in an obese boy at the same camp.

Behavior Therapy in Day Treatment Settings

An example of the use of many of these behavior therapy techniques within the context of day treatment is provided by Risley, Sajwaj, Doke, and Agras (1975), who described a therapeutic day care program for preschoolers with behavior problems. Within a traditional day care activity schedule, they provided for intensive behavioral assessment and intervention with individual children. They reported success with such interventions as

> Time-out contingent upon tantrums, aggressive behavior, cursing, and noncompliance; contingent snacks and privileges for attending to caregivers, appropriate play, proper toileting and dressing, smiling, prolonged attention to tasks, and increasingly complex motor behaviors; differential attention procedures for hyperactive behavior, talking out of turn, sex-appropriate play, mildly disruptive behavior, and crying; overcorrection for certain autistic mannerisms; access to day-care materials contingent upon correct language usage and pre-academic requirements; and a combination of shaping and fading for self-dressing, appropriate play, and self-feeding. (p. 105)

The second format that could be described as a behavioral model of day treatment is one in which all aspects of the day treatment program are organized into a comprehensive contingency management system. Although such a system is usually individualized to some extent, it does provide for standardized application of contingencies to all day treatment patients. This model appears to offer the most potential for efficient use of behavioral techniques in day treatment and is described in detail next.

Comprehensive Contingency Management: The Token Economy

One variety of contingency management system which has been reported to be effective in a number of settings is the token economy (Ayllon & Azrin, 1968). DeVoge and Downey (1975) reported on the application of a token economy to a day treatment program for adolescent and adult psychiatric patients. They first compiled a list of all problematic behaviors being engaged in by program participants. These were then described, clarified, and combined into a workable number of "target behaviors." Observable criteria for reward were then specified for each target behavior. Rewards were given through the use of point booklets in which holes were punched for each point earned by performing at or above criterion for a target behavior. Points were redeemable for privileges, including use of a ward "comfort room," permission to smoke during activity periods, permission to drink coffee anywhere in the building, and freedom to leave the center during lunch. The program was individualized by setting five different "cost" levels for privileges, with all patients starting at the lowest cost level and moving up to the next level upon 2 weeks of criterion behavior. Movement through the rest of the levels was similar, with additional privileges becoming available at each higher level. A further reward was provided by setting a criterion for weekly total point earnings for the group, and if that total was reached or surpassed, the entire group was taken on an outing. Failure to meet the criterion resulted in a group "cleanup" of the center. The results of this token economy program are somewhat difficult to interpret because DeVoge and Downey reported them in terms of cost levels rather than simply across time. However, it appears that there was significant improvement in patients' appearance, punctuality, verbal behavior, and task completion.

Kaufman and O'Leary (1972) established a token economy program for 16 maladjusted adolescents hospitalized in a psychiatric ward. Two classrooms, with 8 students each, were utilized. A positive reinforcement model was used in one classroom. Students were able to earn up to 10 tokens during each of three 15-minute academic periods. Tokens were earned by following basic classroom rules. A response cost model was used in the other classroom. Students were given 10 tokens at the start of each 15-minute academic period. At the end of the period, from zero to 10 tokens were taken back by the teacher for breaking classroom rules. Tokens for each group were redeemable (at a value of 1 cent each) at a ward store that contained a number of items ranging in value from 1 cent to $4. Tokens could be spent each day or accumulated. Results of this program indicated a significant decrease in maladaptive and disruptive behavior under both positive reinforcement and response cost models. The positive reinforcement model appeared slightly more effective than the response cost model.

Mattos, Mattson, Walker, and Buckley (1969) designed a token program in a special classroom for children in fourth, fifth, and sixth grades. These children were (a) hyperactive, (b) abusive toward peers, (c) distractable, (d) defiant, and (e) attentive to academic tasks less than 50% of the time. Academic performance was reinforced by giving points for working on assigned tasks and completing classwork. Points were recorded on a student work card and could be redeemed for free time at a rate of 1 minute per point. The amount of work required per point was initially set at a modest level, and gradually the expectations were raised. A group contingency was also used, with group points exchangeable for a class field trip. Time-out from positive reinforcement and exclusion from school were used to deal with more disruptive behaviors.

Evaluation of this program indicated that children displayed task-oriented behaviors less than 50% of the time prior to treatment.

During the last treatment phase, task-oriented behavior had increased to 84%. A follow-up assessment conducted 2 weeks after the children had returned to their regular classrooms indicated that task-oriented behavior had dropped to 77% of the time, still up 27% from baseline.

McKenzie, Clark, Wolf, Kothera, and Benson (1968) reported on a token reinforcement system in a special class for educationally handicapped children. Recess, free-time activities, permission to be a classroom helper, permission to eat lunch with other children, and teacher praise were all used as reinforcers contingent on academic performance. Children were also given a percentage of their weekly allowance by parents based on their academic performance. Evaluation conducted after the children were returned to regular classrooms indicated that all children but one had improved their academic performance, with the mean score for all subjects increasing from 68% during baseline to 86% following treatment.

Breiling, Shipman, Milligan, and Pepin (1971) used a token system in a classroom of 41 "normal" third-graders without significant behavior problems. Children could earn 15 points per day: 6 for completing assigned academic work, 6 for correctness of completed work, and 3 for demonstrating appropriate social behavior. When a student earned 300 points, he or she was eligible to become a member of the Good Citizenship Council. To remain on the council, a student had to earn a minimum of 12 points a day and demonstrate no inappropriate social behaviors. Regaining council membership once it had been revoked required earning an additional 300 points.

A number of reinforcers accompanied council membership. Members could leave their seats, go to the bathroom, and get a drink of water whenever they desired. They could do their classwork at a special place in the classroom, participate in a special "talk time," and attend council meetings during school. Although no specific evaluation data were presented by the authors, anecdotal evidence suggested that the procedure was effective in enhancing academic and social behavior.

Three studies conducted at a summer camp for emotionally disturbed children (Clements, Willis, & Rickard, 1974; Rickard, Willis, & Clements, 1974; Willis, 1974) all found that tokens made contingent on correct completion of individually programmed academic material resulted in significantly more academic achievement than exposure to the same material without token reinforcers. The tokens in these studies were redeemable for toys and snack foods at a camp store.

One of the most sophisticated and extensively evaluated token programs is the Teaching Family Model devised for delinquent boys and implemented at the Achievement Place group home (Phillips, Phillips, Fixsen, & Wolf, 1973). Although this program has been implemented within the context of a therapeutic group home rather than a day treatment facility, it is still relevant to the design of day treatment token programs. Points are awarded or point fines levied for performance on a wide variety of chores and responsibilities within the home (room cleanup, social interactions, etc.). Children attend public school, and points are given or removed on the basis of teacher evaluations of school performance as communicated on a daily report card that children take to school each day. Points can be exchanged for a variety of privileges, including use of the television, telephone, radio, and record player. Snacks, trips outside the home, and the opportunity to buy clothes and other items can also be chosen. Children carry their own point cards on which are recorded points earned and lost. Every evening, daily points are totaled, and the children's behavior discussed with them. When a child first enters the program, points are exchanged for reinforcers on a daily basis; however, after a period of time, exchanges are made for privileges on a weekly basis. When significant progress has been made, the point system is phased out for that child, and privileges are accorded freely, except when rule violations occurs, much as in the operation of a normal household.

Data comparing the postdischarge behavior of Achievement Place residents with that of delinquents incarcerated at a traditional reform school or placed on probation indicate that Achievement Place youths had fewer police contacts after treatment than either of the other groups. Two years after intervention, 54% of the youths placed on probation and 53% of those sent to reform school had committed delinquent acts resulting in institutionalizations. Only 19% of the Achievement Place residents had been subsequently institutionalized. Three semesters after intervention, 90% of the former Achievement Place residents were still in school, compared to only 9% of those previously sent to reform school and 37% of those who were placed on probation.

THE BREWER-PORCH CHILDREN'S CENTER SYSTEM

The development of a comprehensive contingency management system within the context of a day treatment program for emotionally disturbed children has been accomplished at Brewer-Porch Children's Center at the University of Alabama. In this case, two separate contingency management systems have been established, one for children 7 to 12 years of age with a variety of behavioral and emotional disorders, and one for juvenile-court-referred adolescents served in a separate program.

Young Children's Program

Elementary-school-aged children are served within the context of a 6-hour schoolday. Ten children per classroom engage in a variety of individual and group educational activities under the supervision of a special educational teacher and aide. Much of the academic work is individualized through the use of programmed instructional materials and workbooks. Fifty-five-minute academic periods are interrupted each hour by 5-minute breaks, and snack periods ("juice break") occur twice a day. Children are observed and rated as "on-task" or "off-task" on a rotating interval schedule. Lunch and recreational activities occur outside the classroom. The behavioral program for younger children is based on a levels system, with point earnings determining level placement. There are five levels, with privileges increasing at each level. The following are examples of the differential privileges for each level:

Level 5. At least 92% of the points must be earned the previous week.
1. May be teacher's assistant.
2. May have seconds and the choice of juice at juice break.
3. May serve self at lunch.
4. Can go outside at free time.
5. May have 5 minutes extra at free time.
6. May sharpen pencil and go to the bathroom without permission.

Level 4. Between 86 and 91% of the points must be earned the previous week.
1. May be teacher's assistant.
2. May have seconds and the choice of juice at juice break.
3. May serve self at lunch.
4. May have free time inside.

Level 3. Requires that between 75 and 85% of the points must be earned the previous week.
1. Cannot be teacher's assistant.
2. Cannot have seconds but can have the choice of juice at juice break.

    3. Cannot serve self at lunch.

    4. May have free time inside, in a restricted area.

Level 2. Between 60 and 74% of the points must be earned the previous week.

    1. Cannot be teacher's assistant.

    2. Cannot have seconds or the choice of juice at juice break.

    3. Cannot serve self at lunch.

    4. May have free time inside, in a restricted area, with restricted activities.

Level 1. Less than 60% of the points are earned the previous week.

    1. Cannot be teacher's assistant.

    2. Cannot have juice at juice break.

    3. Cannot serve self at lunch.

    4. May have free time at desk.

In addition to these standard level-based privileges, a wide variety of other privileges, activities, and more tangible rewards can be tailored to an individual child's level. Also, children who have difficulty coping with the weekly interval between level changes can be placed on daily levels until they can tolerate the longer interval.

In this system, the points that determine levels can be earned in several ways, with approximately 300 points available to a child per day. The day is divided into 25 time periods of approximately 15 minutes each. A child can earn between zero and 10 points for how "on-task" (engaging in appropriate behavior) they are during each time period. In addition, children receive between zero and 50 points for their behavior on the van to and from day treatment each day. On-task is defined differently for each activity. Thus, if the classroom activity is arithmetic, being on-task would mean sitting appropriately at the desk with an opened arithmetic book, pencil and paper, and exhibiting classroom-appropriate behavior (e.g., raising hand to talk). Clearly, the criteria would be different during music or free time. Hourly point totals are recorded on "point cards" that children carry at all times. Weekly outings are scheduled at the end of each week for all children earning 80% or more of the points available to them (the number of points available to individual children varies somewhat because of absences, therapy appointments, etc.).

In addition to the previously described point system, children are awarded "cooperation" points for engaging in behaviors that encourage adaptive behaviors or discourage maladaptive behaviors in others. An example would be ignoring another student who is acting silly or helping a child regain his or her temper. Approximately every 5 days, a special activity (movie, slot car racing, etc.) is conducted on an unannounced basis for children who have a criterion number of "co-operation" points. After this activity, the slate is wiped clean, and all children start again with zero "cooperation" points. When certain students are observed to have particular difficulty getting along with each other, a behavioral contract may be established between them so that they can earn two cooperation points for appropriate interactions rather than one. Behavioral contracts can also be negotiated with staff by individual students to earn reinforcers that are otherwise not available.

In conjunction with the point system, "time-out" is used to control disruptive and aggressive behaviors. As a child begins to lose control, the child is informed that he or she is in "time-out" and not earning on-task points. The child is further told that he or she will not be attended to by staff until he or she is on-task again. If the loss of control escalates, the child is taken to the corner of the room with minimum attention or, if necessary, removed to an enclosed time-out room outside the classroom. Children are kept in the time-out room only until they regain behavioral control (usually less than 10 minutes). Before a child leaves any time-out, he or she is required to state what behavior resulted in the time-out and how he or she could have reacted differently. Only after this statement is the child allowed to begin earning on-task points again.

Evaluation of this behavioral day treatment program provides support for its efficacy (Prentice-Dunn, Wilson, & Lyman, 1981). Parent and teacher ratings of problematic behaviors decreased significantly in approximately 85% of the children served in the program. Over three-quarters of enrolled children are able to return to public school classrooms after 1 year in the day treatment program. By comparison, of the children on the waiting list for day treatment because of space limitations, less than 10% are rated as improved after 6 months. Interestingly, children enrolled in the day treatment program are rated at intake as having behavioral problems as severe as those of children enrolled in Brewer-Porch's residential treatment program, although there do appear to be significant differences in family support and resources. There also does not appear to be a significant difference in diagnostic groups between the residential and day treatment referrals. Both groups consist of primarily conduct-disorder and attention-deficit-disorder youngsters, with a minority of anxiety disorders and psychoses. Treatment outcome figures for the residential program are roughly equivalent to those for the day treatment program (Prentice-Dunn, Wilson, & Lyman, 1981).

Adolescent Program

Brewer-Porch's day treatment program for juvenile-court-referred adolescents is structured quite differently from the program for younger children. The basis of the program is points earned through appropriate behavior, but points are not translated into placement on a levels system. Each adolescent can earn a total of 1,700 points each week: (a) 750 points for appropriate behavior in class, at lunch, and on the van; (b) 500 points for academic achievement; (c) 100 points for participating in group therapy; (d) 100 points for participating in individual or family therapy; and (e) 250 points for not cursing. Appropriate behavior points are awarded for meeting operational criteria established for each activity period during the day. Academic achievement is defined as passing a posttest on individualized academic material at the 100% level. Points for participating in therapy sessions are contingent upon attendance and therapists' judgments of seriousness and effort. In most cases, points are awarded on an "all-or-none" basis for a specific area during one activity period.

Earned points may be redeemed for a number of privileges. Students who have earned 80% or more of academic and behavior points during the week are eligible to buy a Friday afternoon outing (movies, skating, etc.). The cost of the trip is set at 80% of possible points that week, so even students who are eligible may not have enough points if they have not participated in therapy, have cursed frequently, or have otherwise received point fines (for property destruction, for instance). Points may also be used to buy time off from school, at a cost of 500 points per hour (and parental permission). A small canteen is also maintained at which students can buy items for consumption during designated breaks.

Representative prices are as follows:

Soft drinks	250 points
Candy bars	150 points
Potato chips	150 points
Brownies	50 points
Cigarettes	500 points per pack

Special order items and outside shopping trips can also be negotiated, with a basic exchange rate of 10 points per penny. Fines of 25 points are attached to each failure to cease an inappropriate behavior upon request, and fines for property destruction are equated to the cost of the damage at the foregoing exchange rate and paid off over a mutually agreed-upon interval (for instance, a 5,000-point fine for

$50 damage paid as a 500-point fine each week for 10 weeks). Serious aggressive episodes, inappropriate sexual conduct, and substance abuse are not dealt with through the contingency system but are treated appropriately in consultation with parents and juvenile court.

Group therapy sessions are largely based on a Rational Emotive Therapy (RET) philosophy (Ellis, 1962) and appear to fit well within the behavioral milieu. Theoretical orientations of individual therapists vary from cognitive behavioral to dynamic, but there appears to be no interference with the process of individual therapy caused by the requirement that the therapist report a judgment as to the client's effort in therapy to the classroom staff.

Outcome evaluation suggests that the adolescent day treatment program is highly effective in reducing behavior problems (Davis, 1978). Only 22% of the youngsters who complete the program (average duration 7 months) have a repeat law violation versus 83% of an untreated, equivalent control group. Only 6% of those completing the program are subsequently placed in a correctional institution versus 20% of the control group. Adolescents entering the program are, on the average, two grade levels behind in academic skills, yet their average gain on achievement test scores from beginning to completion of day treatment is 1.96 months gain for each month in the program.

In summary, therefore, it appears that day treatment is a viable option for treating emotionally and behaviorally disturbed children and adolescents and that a behavioral format for such treatment can be highly effective, even with seriously disturbed youngsters. Further research is required, however, to determine the limitations of this approach and the specific parameters that affect outcome. The advantages of the day treatment approach appear to be significant, and it is imperative that funding agencies and mental health planners be informed of these advantages so that day treatment services are included in a comprehensive continuum of mental health programs for children. It appears that the cost efficiency and treatment effectiveness of behavioral day treatment may be crucial in a future characterized by dwindling public financial resources and increasingly expensive inpatient care.

REFERENCES

Alexander, R. N., Corbett, T. F., & Smigel, J. (1976). The effects of individual and group consequences on school attendance and curfew violations with predelinquent adolescents. *Journal of Applied Behavior Analysis, 9,* 221–226.
Allen, K. E., & Harris, F. R. (1966). Elimination of a child's excessive scratching by

training the mother in reinforcement procedures. *Behavior Research and Therapy, 4,* 79–84.

Altman, K., Haavik, S., & Cook, J. W. (1978). Punishment of self-injurious behavior in natural settings using contingent aromatic ammonia. *Behavior Research and Therapy, 16,* 85–96.

Ayllon, T., & Azrin, N. H. (1968). *The token economy: A motivational system for therapy and rehabilitation.* New York: Appleton-Century-Crofts.

Baumeister, A. A., & Forehand, R. (1972). Effects of contingent shock and verbal command on body rocking of retardates. *Journal of Clinical Psychology, 28,* 586–590.

Bierer, J. (1951). *The day hospital.* London: H. K. Lewis and Company.

Bijou, S. W., & Baer, D. M. (1963). Some methodological contributions from a functional analysis of child development. In L. P. Lipsett & C. S. Spiker (Eds.), *Advances in child development and behavior: Volume 1* (pp. 197–231). New York: Academic Press.

Blinder, B. J., Freeman, D. M., & Stunkard, A. J. (1970). Behavior therapy of anorexia nervosa: Effectiveness of activity as a reenforcer of weight gain. *American Journal of Psychiatry, 126,* 1093–1098.

Blom, G. E., Farley, G. K., & Ekanger, C. (1973). A psycho-educational treatment program: Its characteristics and results. In G. E. Blom & G. K. Farley (Eds.), *Report on activities of the Day Care Center of the University of Colorado Medical Center to the Commonwealth Foundation* (pp. 65–81). Denver: University of Colorado Medical Center Press.

Brandsma, J. M., & Stein, L. I. (1973). The use of punishment as a treatment modality: A case report. *Journal of Nervous and Mental Disease, 156,* 30–37.

Breiling, J. P., Shipman, H., Milligan, J., & Pepin, L. (1971). Glugies, snirkles, and models: Three systems of token reinforcement in the grade school classroom. *Educational Technology Research, 14,* 1–20.

Cameron, D. E. (1947). The day hospital. *Medical Hospital, 69,* 3.

Clark, D. F. (1966). Behavior therapy of Gilles de la Tourette's syndrome. *British Journal of Psychiatry, 112,* 771–778.

Clark, H. B., Greene, B. F., Macrae, J. W., McNees, M. P., Davis, J. L., & Risley, T. R. (1977). A parent advice package for family shopping trips: Development and evaluation. *Journal of Applied Behavior Analysis, 10,* 605–624.

Clements, C. B., Willis, J. W., & Rickard, H. C. (1974). Schoolhouse in the woods: A first attempt. In H. C. Rickard & M. Dinoff (Eds.), *Behavior modification in children: Case studies and illustrations from a summer camp* (pp. 132–147). Tuscaloosa: The University of Alabama Press.

Conway, J. B., & Bucher, B. D. (1974). "Soap in the mouth" as an aversive consequence. *Behavior Therapy, 5,* 154–156.

Davis, J. C. (1978). Community intensive treatment for youth. *Alabama Law Enforcement Planning Agency Grant Proposal* (No. 78-A2-10), Montgomery, AL.

DeVoge, J. T., & Downey, W. E., Jr. (1975). A token economy program in a community mental health day treatment center. In W. D. Gentry (Ed.), *Applied behavior modification* (pp. 84–108). St. Louis: C. V. Mosby Company.

Dinoff, M., Rickard, H. C., & Colwick, J. (1974). Weight reduction through successive contracts. In H. C. Rickard & M. Dinoff (Eds.), *Behavior modification in children: Case studies and illustrations from a summer camp* (pp. 104–109). Tuscaloosa: University of Alabama Press.

Dinoff, M., Serum, C., & Rickard, H. C. (1974). Controlling rebellious behavior through successive contracts. In H. C. Rickard & M. Dinoff (Eds.), *Behavior modifi-*

cation in children: Case studies and illustrations from a summer camp (pp. 115–122). Tuscaloosa: University of Alabama Press.

Doty, D. W., McInnis, T., & Paul, G. L. (1974). Remediation of negative side effects of an ongoing response-cost system with chronic mental patients. *Journal of Applied Behavior Analysis, 7,* 191–198.

Drabman, R. S., & Spitalnik, R. (1973). Social isolation as a punishment procedure: A controlled study. *Journal of Experimental Child Psychology, 16,* 236–249.

Ellis, A. (1962). *Reason and emotion in psychotherapy.* New York: Lyle Stewart.

Epstein, L. H., Doke, L. A., Sajwaj, T. E., Sorrell, S., & Rimmer, B. (1974). Generality and side effects of overcorrection. *Journal of Applied Behavior Analysis, 7,* 385–390.

Foxx, R. M., & Azrin, N. H. (1973). The elimination of autistic self-stimulatory behavior by overcorrection. *Journal of Applied Behavior Analysis, 6,* 1–14.

Freedman, A. M. (1959). Day hospitals for severely disturbed schizophrenic children. *American Journal of Psychiatry, 115,* 893–898.

Gelfand, D. M., & Hartmann, D. P. (1975). *Child behavior analysis and therapy.* New York: Pergamon Press.

Goldfarb, W., Goldfarb, N., & Pollack, R. C. (1966). Treatment of childhood schizophrenia: A three year comparison of day and residential treatment. *Archives of General Psychiatry, 14,* 119–128.

Hamilton, J., & Standahl, J. (1969). Suppression of stereotyped screaming behavior in a profoundly retarded institutionalized female. *Journal of Experimental Child Psychology, 7,* 114–121.

Harris, S. L., & Romanczyk, R. (1976). Treating self-injurious behavior of a retarded child by overcorrection. *Behavior Therapy, 7,* 235–239.

Homme, L. (1970). *How to use contingency contracting in the classroom.* Champaign, IL: Research Press.

Homme, L. E., DeBaca, P. C., Devine, J. V., Steinhorst, R., & Rickert, E. J. (1963). Use of the Premack Principle in controlling the behavior of nursery school children. *Journal of the Experimental Analysis of Behavior, 6,* 544.

Kaufman, K. F., & O'Leary, K. D. (1972). Reward, cost, and self-evaluation procedures for disruptive adolescents in a psychiatric hospital school. *Journal of Applied Behavior Analysis, 5,* 293–309.

Kazdin, A. E. (1973). The effect of response cost and aversive stimulation in suppressing punished and nonpunished speech disfluencies. *Behavior Therapy, 4,* 73–82.

Lahey, B. B., McNees, M. P., & McNees, M. C. (1973). Control of an obscene "verbal tic" through timeout in an elementary school classroom. *Journal of Applied Behavioral Analysis, 6,* 101–104.

LaVietes, R. L., Cohen, R., Reens, R., & Ronall, R. (1965). Day treatment center and school: Seven years experience. *American Journal of Orthopsychiatry, 35,* 160–169.

Lovaas, O. I., & Simmons, J. Q. (1969). Manipulation of self-destruction in three retarded children. *Journal of Applied Behavior Analysis, 2,* 143–157.

Lovaas, O. I., Frietag, G., Kinder, M. I., Rubenstein, B. D., Schaeffer, B., & Simmons, J. Q. (1966). Establishment of social reinforcers in two schizophrenic children on the basis of food. *Journal of Experimental Child Psychology, 4,* 109–125.

Madsen, C. K., & Madsen, C. H., Jr. (1972). *Parents/children/discipline: A positive approach.* Boston: Allyn & Bacon.

Madsen, C. H., Jr., Becker, W. C., Thomas, D. R., Koser, L., & Plager, E. (1968). An analysis of the reinforcing function of "sit down" commands. In R. K. Parker (Ed.), *Readings in educational psychology* (pp. 265–278). Boston: Allyn & Bacon.

Mattos, R. L., Mattson, R. H., Walker, H. M., & Buckley, N. K. (1969). Reinforcement and aversive control in the modification of behavior. *Academic Therapy, 5,* 37–52.

McKenzie, H. S., Clark, M., Wolf, M. M., Kothera, R., & Benson, C. (1968). Behavior modification of children with learning disabilities using grades as tokens and allowances as backup reinforcers. *Exceptional Children, 34,* 745–752.

O'Leary, K. D., Kaufman, K. F., Kass, R., & Drabman, R. (1970). The effects of loud and soft reprimands on the behavior of disruptive students. *Exceptional Children, 37,* 145–155.

Phillips, E. L., Phillips, E. A., Fixsen, D. L., & Wolf, M. M. (1973). Behavior shaping works for delinquents. *Psychology Today, 7,* 75–79.

Premack, D. (1965). Reinforcement theory. In D. Levine (Ed.), *Nebraska Symposium on Motivation* (pp. 123–180). Lincoln: University of Nebraska Press.

Prentice-Dunn, S., Wilson, D. R., & Lyman, R. D. (1981). Client factors related to outcome in a residential and day treatment program for children. *Journal of Clinical Child Psychology, 10,* 188–191.

Redl, F. (1966). *When we deal with children.* New York: Free Press.

Rickard, H. C., Willis, J. W., & Clements, C. B. (1974). Effects of contingent and noncontingent token reinforcement upon classroom performance. In H. C. Rickard & M. Dinoff (Eds.), *Behavior modification in children: Case studies and illustrations from a summer camp* (pp. 115–122). Tuscaloosa: University of Alabama Press.

Risley, T. R. (1968). The effects and side effects of punishing the autistic behaviors of a deviant child. *Journal of Applied Behavior Analysis, 1,* 21–34.

Risley, T., Sajwaj, T., Doke, L., & Agras, S. (1975). Specialized day care as a psychiatric outpatient service. In E. Ramp & G. Semb (Eds.), *Behavioral analysis: Areas of research & application* (pp. 97–123). Englewood Cliffs, NJ: Prentice-Hall.

Sajwaj, T., Libet, J., & Agras, S. (1974). Lemon-juice therapy: The control of life-threatening rumination in a six-month-old infant. *Journal of Applied Behavior Analysis, 7,* 557–563.

Sanok, R. L., & Striefel, S. (1979). Elective mutism: Generalization of verbal responding across people and settings. *Behavior Therapy, 10,* 357–371.

Stone, M. C. (1970). Behavior shaping in a classroom for children with cerebral palsy. *Exceptional Children, 36,* 674–677.

Stuart, R. B. (1974). Behavioral contracting within the families of delinquents. In O. I. Lovaas & B. D. Bucher (Eds.), *Perspectives in behavior modification with deviant children* (pp. 319–335). Englewood Cliffs, NJ: Prentice-Hall.

Swan, W. W., & Wood, M. M. (1976). Making decisions about treatment. In M. M. Wood (Ed.), *Developmental therapy.* Baltimore: University Park Press.

Tahmisian, J. A., & McReynolds, W. T. (1971). Use of parents as behavioral engineers in the treatment of a school phobic girl. *Journal of Counseling Psychology, 18,* 225–228.

Tate, B. G., & Baroff, G. S. (1966). Aversive control of self-injurious behavior in a psychotic boy. *Behaviour Research and Therapy, 4,* 281–287.

Walton, D. (1961). Experimental psychology and the treatment of a ticquer. *Journal of Child Psychology and Psychiatry, 2,* 148–155.

Walton, D. (1964). Massed practice and simultaneous reduction in drive level: Further evidence of the efficacy of this approach to the treatment of tics. In H. J. Eysenck (Ed.), *Experiments in behavior therapy* (pp. 398–400). Oxford, England: Pergamon Press.

Wielkiewicz, R. M. (1986). *Behavior management in the schools: Principles and procedures.* New York: Pergamon Press.

Willis, J. W. (1974). Contingent token reinforcement in an educational program for emotionally disturbed children. In H. C. Rickard and M. Dinoff (Eds.), *Behavior modification in children: Case studies and illustrations from a summer camp* (pp. 157–169). Tuscaloosa: University of Alabama Press.

Wilson, D. R., & Lyman, R. D. (1982). Time-out in the treatment of childhood behavior problems: Implementation and research issues. *Child and Family Behavior Therapy, 4,* 5–20.

Wood, M. M. (Ed.). (1975). *Developmental therapy: A textbook for teachers as therapists for emotionally disturbed young children.* Baltimore: University Park Press.

Zang, L. C. (1978). The antisocial aggressive school age child: Day hospitals. In B. B. Wolman, J. Egan, & A. O. Ross (Eds.), *Handbook of treatment of mental disorders in childhood and adolescence* (pp. 317–329). Englewood Cliffs, NJ: Prentice-Hall.

Zimet, S. G., & Farley, G. K. (1985). Day treatment for children in the United States. *Journal of the American Academy of Child Psychiatry, 24,* 732–738.

Zimet, S. G., Farley, G. K., Silver, J., Hebert, F. B., Robb, E. D., Ekanger, C., & Smith, D. (1980). Behavior and personality changes in emotionally disturbed children enrolled in a psychoeducational day treatment center. *Journal of the American Academy of Child Psychiatry, 19,* 240–256.

7

The Application of Psychodynamic Principles to Day Treatment

C. JANET NEWMAN

INTRODUCTION

Psychodynamic Principles

Psychodynamic principles refer to broad applications of findings gained from psychoanalysis and psychoanalytic psychotherapy of adults and children. In addition, direct observations of infants in families, as well as longitudinal studies of individuals, have immensely expanded the body of psychodynamic knowledge. *A Psychiatric Glossary* (American Psychiatric Association, 1975, p. 127) offers this definition:

> Psychodynamics: The systematized knowledge and theory of human behavior and its motivation, the study of which depends largely upon the functional significance of emotion. Psychodynamics recognizes the role of *unconscious* motivation in human behavior. It is a predictive science, based on the assumption that a person's total make-up and probable reactions at any given moment are the product of past interactions between his specific genetic endowment and the environment in which he has lived since conception.

C. JANET NEWMAN • Department of Psychiatry, College of Medicine, University of Cincinnati, Cincinnati, Ohio 45267.

Essential Elements of Day Treatment

Westman (1979) outlined the essential day program elements as being the therapeutic milieu, psychotherapy, specialized educational services, family therapy, parent liaison, recreational therapy, craft, art and music therapy, language therapy, community liaison, psychopharmacology, the health consultation system, and staff development. In this outline of psychodynamic principles we shall refer often to these programmatic aspects where psychodynamic processes occur.

Principles of Psychodynamic Day Treatment

The goal of this chapter is to conceptualize several basic psychodynamic principles and to use vignettes or illustrations from some of the program elements listed before. These examples come from my 17 years of experience as Medical Director of the Elementary Day Treatment Program at the Children's Psychiatric Center of the Jewish Hospital of Cincinnati. Day treatment has been a major treatment modality in this center since 1970, when a new wing containing day treatment classrooms was added to the inpatient building. Since then, under the leadership of Othilda Krug, there have been four to eight classes of seven children each for preschool and elementary-aged children. The Children's Psychiatric Center has always been affiliated with the Division of Child and Adolescent Psychiatry of the Department of Psychiatry of the University of Cincinnati. The psychodynamic principles described will be (a) unconscious motivation, (b) mental structuring, (c) self and object relations, (d) transference and countertransference, and (e) specific dynamic significance of *day* treatment. All of these principles interact constantly and simultaneously in a psychodynamic day treatment setting. The first three principles, however, are based on findings that have been developed in depth over a period of historical time that allowed for increased understanding and shifts of emphasis. They have evolved from one to the other, and, in my experience are most clearly understood in this evolutionary conceptual perspective.

UNCONSCIOUS MOTIVATION

The concept of the unconscious is the sine qua non of a psychodynamic orientation. Freud first described the existence of an unconscious in his studies of slips of speech and actions, (1901); infantile sexuality, (1905a); jokes, (1905b); and transference and countertransference (1910). These discoveries were made possible by Freud's clinical method of total listening to his patients' free associations, free as much as possible from selection and control. Like the microscope that opened up a new world of microorganisms, the invention of listening carefully to everything a patient said and did opened up a new vista of depth psychological patterns of which a patient was, at the time, totally unaware. What was thought of as the dynamic unconscious was kept that way by clinically observable resistance or defensiveness, which came to be conceptualized as repression. The contents of the dynamic unconscious were unacceptable wishes, which were seen as in conflict with the conscious mind.

To exemplify the role of unconscious motivations affecting learning, a day treatment patient's dream will be described. A highly intelligent 10-year-old girl diagnosed as overanxious disorder was very frightened by her frequent fantasies of the imminent deaths of her parents. She was bright but very inhibited in school. In psychotherapy she reported the following dream. "I dreamt of an old man dead. He was born in 1499. They don't live so long since Columbus discovered America." This was the entire dream. She commented that the dream felt silly, scary, and awful. Her thoughts about the number 1499 led her to recall that 14 was her male cousin's age and that the family had celebrated his birthday the previous weekend. Her father, however, had to work during this celebration, and this had made her very angry, which led to more fantasies of his death. When asked about the 99, she became thoughtful, adding her parents' ages, arriving at 91 as the sum. Recalling her cousin's birthday again, she remembered that she used to sleep in bed with him when they were both much younger. She then drew a square, writing 99 within it, explaining this was also like her mom and dad in bed. She had wanted to marry her cousin when they were grown-ups, but the bishop said cousins could never marry. This warning had made her feel terrible, guilty, and excited. She hesitantly explained that she and her cousin had touched each other's bodies, and she had discovered a new part of his body she had never seen or felt before.

When her psychiatrist later talked with her teacher, it was learned that the class was currently discussing the discovery by Columbus of America in 1492. Her teacher reported that a map involving the Atlantic coastline of the new continent had greatly excited her. He explained that she had been especially fascinated and overstimulated by Florida. She had had problems, not only with geography, but with the shapes of certain numerals and letters earlier in her education, which had puzzled her previous teachers.

These clinical facts, including her dreams, were very useful for the clinical team working with her. The child psychiatrist explained to her that as she learned letters, numerals, and geographical shapes, it was easy to understand how some of these might look like parts of her body or her cousin's. When she saw the similarities, she might feel "scared," "awful and silly" (to use her own words). She was helped to talk more directly and easily about her body and her ideas and feelings about sex. Her need to endow school material with inner fantasies was diminished by the therapist's encouragement of her free, more direct, and independent expression of her curiosities and fantasies about male and female bodies. With this increasingly free verbalization, she was far less inclined to use school material as a projection of her inner conflicts and drives.

These clinical data, shared with her teacher, facilitated his increasing patience and empathy with the early errors this child and other patients made in their initial attempts to read, to calculate, and later to understand more difficult concepts.

This kind of interdisciplinary sharing helped teachers to see, in a more general way, how children often saw the concrete imagery of their earliest exposure to letters and numerals like Chinese pictograms, like tiny pictures that had strong similarities to emotionally laden shapes with which they were preoccupied in this 5- to 7-year-old stage. The staff knew that later, as children's understanding of letters became less connected with shape and more connected with sounds, they could deal with a higher level of abstraction that would facilitate their ability to read.

For teachers who had chosen to work in psychodynamic day treatment centers, this kind of clinical explanation often made a lot of sense. For others who were less psychoanalytically interested, it was often seen as overly picky, bodily centered, and even ridiculous. A few teachers could later admit they had privately thought the psychiatrists' ideas were silly.

A day treatment program, however, offers a constant flow of examples in learning, cognition, and teaching processes that come under the sway of the child's primitive and unconscious mind, and these examples become very convincing to the clinical teachers who work for years in such a setting.

Such examples used in psychodynamic seminars for public-school teachers often meet with instant recognition and insight. One such teacher described a child who avoided sharply pointing his capital A's and K's because he said these were "sharp like weapons" and made him scared.

A day treatment program has the potential of being used as a natural laboratory for the discovery of many linkages between inner drives, self-concepts, fantasies, and conflicts with basic issues in learning, including not only learning problems but surprising successes in learning and creativity.

Many psychoanalytic authors such as Berlin and Szurek (1965), Bettelheim and Zelan (1982), Blom (1979), Hirschberg (1953), Newman, Dember, and Krug (1973), Pearson (1954), and Rosen (1955) have discussed the enormous impact of unconscious factors on learning situations.

THE STRUCTURAL MODEL, OR "THE STRUCTURE OF THE PSYCHE"

The original differentiation of the mind into conscious and unconscious components came to be referred to as "the topographic model", using a mapping out or location metaphor for mental functions. Such metaphors were meant to guide our concepts but not to be taken literally. Clinical samples illustrating this model were given in the previous section.

After this profound discovery, further psychoanalytic explorations led Freud to describe more complex interrelating mental functions. In 1923, he wrote *Ego and the Id*. In his original German, this was *Das Ich und Das Es*, which might more vividly and emotionally be translated in English as "The I and the It" (Bettelheim, 1982). In this publication, he also added the *Uber-Ich*, or *superego*; again, in plain English, the *Over-I* watches over, judges, punishes, rewards, and loves the ego or the *I*. This differentiation of the mind into three major functions or agencies was deeply relevant to a wide range of human conflicts and difficulties. This became known as *the structural model*. Basic issues brought out in the simpler *topographic model* were not dropped out; they remained vital. For example, the id was totally unconscious and could only be known by its derivatives such as dreams, slips, or symptoms, which erupted into the ego. Both the ego and superego had conscious and unconscious components. For example, many of the ego's defensive functions protecting it from anxiety were unconscious. The id contained the repressed memories and disowned drives that the ego had to implement in an acceptable way or to master or defend itself against. The superego would, from a different perspective, unconsciously observe these interactions and generate feelings of goodness, virtue, self-esteem or wrongdoing, shame or guilt, emotional consequences felt in the ego. The superego was a later development, acquired as the infant grew older, and was made up by values and attitudes of the parents that had been absorbed or internalized unconsciously as the child's superego.

All these concepts (topographic, unconscious, conscious, structural, ego, id, superego) appear more concrete than they were meant to be. Mental processes are hard to understand and categorize. Analogies or metaphors, although aiding our understanding, may be taken so literally that they block further understanding. Freud and the early analysts were trying to describe profound mental discoveries, by pre-existing terminology (which was loaded with other meanings) or invent new terminologies as metaphors. Such terminology then had to undergo extremely variable and difficult translations influenced by the culture and language of the translators. We will feel lucky if we have sketched it out without too much confusion.

PEREMPTORY DRIVES

The peremptory drives (originally sexual, later, also aggressive) produced conflicts in the ego resulting in anxiety and guilt, both of which evoked defense mechanisms. These, if chronic or intense, could be pathogenic. Brenner (1955) elucidated that a drive in humans, in contrast to instincts in animals, did not include the motor response but only the central excitation. The motor activity was mediated by the ego. The typical motor behaviors of an individual in response to inner drives were learned in the context of the child's environment. The drives produced cycles of tension and satiation. Each drive had a source, an aim, an impetus, and an object. The object (which could be animate or inanimate) existed primarily for the satisfaction of the drive according to the pleasure principle. The sexual drives developed in successive stages, proceeding from the newborn's oral dependent satisfactions and later oral aggressivity to the anal phase when defecation was accompanied by sensual pleasure to the older child's interests in the phallus and its presence or absence in boys or girls. Later differential interests in mothers by boys, and fathers by girls, represented a basic sexual landmark known as the oedipal stage. Superego development prevented inappropriate physical contacts, and a subsequent period of latency set in, which was relatively drive quiescent and a good period for learning.

At the time of its publication in 1905, this smooth erotic developmental sequence met with shock and derision. Today we would place it among a wide number of developmental lines (Freud, A., 1965).

The power of sexuality is no longer denied. From a developmental perspective, even prior to pregnancy, parental expectations include a range from high hopes to bitter disappointments and critical decisions. Many young women experience this quite alone, as do the possible impregnating young men. Parents fantasize intensely about the developing fetus, as they make crucial choices about names, type of delivery, method of feeding, and so on.

The actual sex of the newborn infant is often pronounced and welcomed with a range of stirring and profound emotions: "It's a boy!", "It's a girl!", with unending echoes of joy, glee, satisfaction or disappointment, even rejection, which have lifelong influences on subsequent gender identity, sexual development, and future partner choice.

Besides the physiological consequences of an infant's sex, the latter is already influencing parents' attitudes in feeding, cuddling, and playing. These primary interactions have much to do with later patterns of yearnings for affection and intimacy.

Toddlers become gradually or suddenly aware of the emotionally startling anatomical differences of the sexes, leading to a variety of reactions.

At the same time in development, issues of socialization of the excretory functions are not unrelated to sexual development because the organs of excretion are intricately interwoven with those of sexuality, even more so in the mind of the child. Parental attitudes to the region generally may include pleasure, disgust, overstimulation, or lack of consistent care in diapering and later toilet training.

Later, children and their parents are anxious about discussions of sex. Children sense the tension and often turn to each other for answers. Masturbation has both soothing and disconcerting conflictual meanings, accompanied by fantasies lasting well into adolescence and beyond.

Adolescents face the realization that sex is now something they can begin to do, and this is a source of conflict within themselves, with their parents and in society. Concerns about attractiveness, sexual functioning, pregnancy, and disease accompany the adaptation to sudden growth and new secondary sexual characteristics.

Adults are concerned with marital or alternative relationships and with the vicissitudes of orgasm and reproduction. The integration of love and sex is a tantalizing goal not always achieved.

Responsiveness to parenthood and a new cycle of generations arouses a great range of emotions. The functions of fatherhood as well as motherhood are undergoing change.

Sexuality is the subject of major psychological and medical studies. It is a major theme of religions, cultures, art, poetry, drama, and literature. Sexuality is a major, if sometimes hidden, component in commerce and advertising. Its role in criminal activities, abuse, family breakdown, divorce, custody disputes, is endless and well known to mental health professionals.

The interrelationships of sexuality, narcissism, territoriality, aggression, and competition are complex. In expansive political terms, these may take the form of violence and group-sanctioned combat. Freud was bold in bringing the psychology of mucoid midline zones, apertures, and protuberances into the generalized conations, cognitions, perceptions, apperceptions, and emotions of an earlier psychology.

Manifestations of Sexuality and Aggression in Day Treatment

By observing childhood manifestations of sexuality and aggressivity in a day treatment setting, the staff is only too aware of urinations that have intentionally missed the toilet bowl, graffiti on the bathroom walls, sexual activities by children seizing a moment when an adult's back is turned, obscene gestures done to the currently scapegoated child, playing the "dozens" about each other's mother, and probably a new game about fathers. Some children are truly baffled by this mysterious creation of themselves and how it happens. Adopted children are often told things in a special tone of voice. Some children abuse each other and the staff just as they have been abused. They are aggressive through words, through hitting, or with a knife. They physically attack each other or the staff, expressing by their behaviors some form of aggressivity (displacing hurts or rage in the family), which may be threatening and anxiety producing to the day treatment staff, worrying about the safety of the children.

EGO CONCEPTS

Turning now to ego concepts, Anna Freud (1936) elaborated a number of defense mechanisms elicited by anxiety. Such defenses have been succinctly listed by Brenner (1955) as repression, suppression, and reaction formation, isolation, undoing, denial, projection, turning against the self, introjection, identification, and regression. Hartmann (1939) totally reformulated the concept of the ego to be far more comprehensive than its defensive functions. He postulated that the ego was not only defensive but adaptive to the environment. He defined the functions of the ego as intelligence, perception, memory, synthesis, impulse delay, talent and creativity, and many others, each of which goes through its own development. Hartmann, Kris, and Loewenstein (1946) became known as the creators of ego psychology, and much more emphasis was, from then on, placed on ego development. A contemporary listing of ego functions (Bernstein & Warner, 1981) includes, in addition to those mentioned, motor function, judgment, perception, cognition, concentration, abstraction, learning, reasoning, attention, recall, recognition, retention, memory, imagination, and the capacity for fantasy formation. We must add reality testing, modulation of affect, tension control, altruism, humor, anticipation, and sublimation. Other ego functions include novelty seeking, curiosity, exploratory behavior, mastery, integration, and synthesis.

Is every mental function an ego function? The answer to this is not simple. Those so-called ego functions that are generally conflict free and adaptive might be more simply labeled as *mental functions*. A good example is a well-known cluster of functions (mental or ego) that develop in toddlerhood: locomotion, speech, and toilet control. In terms of psychoanalytic developmental psychology, it was considered that locomotion is more conflict free than speech, which in turn is more conflict free than toilet control. Thus it might have been logical to place the mastery of locomotion and its mental consequences in a list of *mental functions*. Mahler and her coworkers (1975), however, have clearly shown that a toddler's early walking is deeply involved in processes of separation and individuation in relation to mother. Some toddlers cling anxiously, and others feel free to roam, explore, walk, and run, confident of occasional checking back with mother or using their equally new voices to call out to her.

Especially for emotionally disturbed children, many of their so-called *mental functions* may have developed deficiently, often later to become involved in conflicts. Or, alternatively, some of their mental functions may have been conflicted in their early development.

Any deficiency in *mental functions*, as it becomes recognized by the parents or teachers, is threatening to the family. The task of teasing-out innate environmental and unconscious factors in learning disabilities or attention deficit disorders is formidable. When a problem is considered to be organic, this does not mean that it has no unconscious or conflictual ramifications. In fact, such problems are often accompanied by more unconscious conflict and pain, rather than less. Organic and psychodynamic factors work together, synergistically with "both-and" consequences rather than "either-or."

It is important to remember that *ego function* does not imply pathology for that function. It is also important to realize that broadly understood *mental functions* do not imply freedom from unconscious processes.

The work of ego psychologists has made possible the integration of developmental cognitive findings from nonanalytic psychologists such as Piaget (1936). Anthony (1956, 1957) has been instrumental in linking Piaget's cognitive stages with psychodynamic stages.

Therapeutic Applications of Mental Structuring

A day treatment program must imbue all the elements listed by Westman with qualities that build ego structure. The therapeutic milieu he listed first is a term borrowed from well-established total residential programs such as those of Bettelheim and Sylvester (1948), Bettelheim (1950), Krug (1952), Redl and Wineman (1957), Szurek, Berlin, and Boatman (1971), and Trieshman, Whittaker, and Brendtro (1969). The psychodynamic guidelines for therapeutic and pleasant mealtimes are especially relevant for day treatment lunchtimes. Managing meals, responding to demands for thirds, or guiding the child who smears his or her food are important issues. Specific psychodynamic guidelines are needed to integrate individual differences in managing a lunchtime therapeutic milieu.

Other examples of psychodynamic guidelines are those required for appropriate and nonpunitive management of the child who is out of control. The staff needs to share a methodolgy and feel confident with it, and Redl's phrase *what to do until the ego comes* is a good one. His techniques of the life space interview and time-outs are creative and useful. Equally important are quiet rooms with punching bags or special areas where a child can sit and reflectively restore equilibrium or talk with staff who can respond to feelings with empathic and supportive understanding.

In group therapy and individual psychotherapy, children learn to verbalize and articulate their own feelings and interactions with others, as well as develop insights and controls around problem behaviors. The role of verbalization in conscious self-observation is an ego function vital in therapy. Children in creative writing, music, and art therapy learn the gratifications and creative pleasures that can be obtained through sublimation and mastery. A milieu, through its people, programs, structures, atmosphere, color, and concern, must be, in Winnicott's words, "a facilitating environment" (1965).

SELF AND OBJECT RELATIONS

Although the structural theory described is a valuable one-person psychology, it does not begin to describe this person's development. In Winnicott's famous phrase, "There is no such thing as a baby . . . one sees a nursing couple" (1952). He added, "Without a good enough technique of infant care the new human being has no chance whatever." Infant–mother (or caretaker) relationships are vital for survival and healthy ego development. Over a span of years, each minute of interpersonal exchange becomes internalized as part of the child's own mental structures. The child identifies with his or her parents. As the child matures physically and neurologically, he or she yearns to do what the parents do, and especially what they do for the child. For example, when mother feeds her child with a spoon, as soon as the child is able, he or she will grab it, saying with glee, "*Me* do it!" Idealization, identification, and internalization are processes whereby parents' and others' mental functions become part of the child's. In addition, the child forms ever more complex images of them as vital people, or "objects," while building up self-experiences into increasing firmer images of himself or herself as a "self," with a gender, identity, qualities that are the child's own. The child's self-identity reminds us of the forceful *das Ich* or *the I* of Freud's earlier terminology. Such powerful mental images become connected with sounds with the exciting onset of speech.

It is significant that although the more or less smooth developmental patterns of identification and internalization are the products of relating day in and day out to usually empathic and concerned parents, historically, much of the crucial nature of parent–child relations was picked up in seriously defective, pathological environments. It is often the case that we learn about health from illness. For example, Spitz was a pioneer child analyst who made observational studies of babies and their caretakers in different settings that occur in natural society. Anna Freud has called such studies "experiments in nature." Spitz (1945, 1946; Spitz & Cobliner, 1965) found that babies in the affectionate care of their imprisoned delinquent mothers developed physically and emotionally far better than those in a foundling home where technically antiseptic nurses on different shifts took excellent physical care of the babies. He also described the severe depression that develops in infants who have experienced several months of separation from their mothers in the latter part of their first year of life. He later outlined major stages of object-related developments, such as the "smiling response" around 2 to 3 months, separation anxiety at 7 to 9 months, as well as linguistic developments, including saying "no" in the second year of life.

Other studies include those by Harlow (1958) who compared the relationships of infant monkeys to artificial mothers, some equipped with a bottle and others covered with terry cloth. This experiment showed that the monkeys who thrived and later become capable of adult relatedness were those who obtained sensual closeness to the terry-cloth mothers. This experiment showed that orality was not the powerful drive Freud had postulated, at least not for monkeys. Affectionate physical contact and clinging were more powerful.

In 1969, John Bowlby published a book entitled *Attachment,* in which he stressed that sucking, clinging, following, crying, and smiling are all vital parts of attachment behavior, which he defined as a general "built-in propensity" of infants. Bowlby was very impressed by ethologists who had studied relationships among animals in nature.

Winnicott (1953) recognized the intensity of the mother–infant relationship and developed the profound concept of the "transitional object" (the teddy bears or special blanket known to most mothers) that represents a bridge between mother and infant when mother is not immediately available. These transitional objects are both *me* and *not me* for the infant and are clutched by infants in the absence of their mothers as symbols of mother. Winnicott further speculated that his transitional area or space between psychic reality and external reality, or between child and mother, was a region involved in child play, child therapy, and even human culture, the arts, and religions.

Mahler and colleagues (1975) was the outstanding psychoanalyst who systematically observed and studied infants from birth to age 3 in mother/infant pairs in a nursery. She described the concept of separation–individuation, with its subphases of gratifying symbiosis, differentiation, and enthusiastic practicing. She also noted the formation of remembered mental images, which were later connected with words, and the emotional realization of smallness, helplessness, and dependency, which she called the phase of rapprochement characterized by the infant's yearning again for closeness with mother. Finally, the well-remembered and dependable mother (the *internal representation of mother*) ushered in the phase of object constancy upon which the child can rely for hours or a few days, whether angry or loving, and while in nursery school or day care (Fraiberg, 1969).

The role of the father has received greatly heightened attention by some writers. Abelin (1971) stressed the major contributions of the father during the practicing subphase. Cath, Gurwitt, and Ross (1982) edited a fundamental psychodynamic collection of papers on vital father–child relationships. Greenspan (1982) described the father as *the second other.* Herzog described a special kind of night terror in toddlers yearning for absent fathers (1980). He also vividly differentiated the behaviors of fathers toward young daughters and young sons (1984). He pointed out that the birth order of boys and girls is an important factor in their sexual identity development.

Roiphe and Galenson have reviewed the development of sexual identities in toddler boys and girls (1981). They stated that the infant's recognition of sexual differences, accompanied by anxieties and depressions, can be observed as early as 17 months and occurs concurrently with symbol, language, and fantasy development. Solnit and Neubauer (1986) have connected object constancy with both the dyadic mother–infant relationship and early triadic relations with two different kinds of parents. Even in a one-parent family (frequent in day treatment programs), the yearned-for or frustrating psychological presence of the absent parent influences the child. In the older child there is, in addition, a sexual constellation of feelings toward the parent of the opposite sex and competitive feelings toward the parent of the same sex. These are the later intense emotions of the oedipal period from 3 to 6, in which parents and siblings, as Anthony (1970) noted, are caught up as well. Sarnoff (1976) and also Shapiro and Perry (1976) have redefined the so-called latency period, when the elementary-school-aged child is capable of appearing relatively quiescent, compliant, and ready for school.

Therapeutic Applications of Self and Object Relations

In a day treatment setting, children and parents undertake the exposure of psychopathological self and object relations, with the hope of obtaining therapeutic resolution of deep family conflicts. The staff of a day treatment center is composed of adults who have chosen to work professionally, through psychiatry, psychology, social work, and special education, with children and their families. Knowing in depth some aspect of human (or object) relations, they are, through psychodynamic psychotherapy and psychodynamic education, offering new relationships to each child in the program and each parent who can participate.

Mark was a 9-year-old boy with a diagnosis of borderline syndrome. He was extremely depressed during and following the loss of his father through divorce. Mark's teacher in the day treatment program observed Mark's difficulties with reading comprehension and his low achievement test scores. Mark was unable to understand the meanings of paragraphs despite good phonetic skills. His arithmetic was also below the level expected considering his intelligence. He was disorganized, impulsive, and depressed. Because of mother's views of her ex-husband's problems, she did not allow frequent visitation or made sure it was supervised by one of the father's family members. Because the mother had initiated treatment for her son's symptoms, the boy's father was initially suspicious and anxious about any connection with the day treatment program. However, the child's therapist was vigorous in pursuing a contact with him, and eventually a response was forthcoming. The father at first was cautious in expressing his feelings about the treatment situation or his son's problems. He had disagreed with the mother's search for help. The child's therapist was consistent in making appointments with him, and the father began to give voice to his own feelings and perspectives. Eventually, the therapist decided to see father and son together (with custodial mother's consent), as a type of familial therapy. At first, the father and son were timid and cautious with each other. The therapist engaged them in emotion-laden conversation and some three-way games. Father grew more animated as he began to enjoy the playfulness of his son and himself in the company of a woman therapist. He said this made him feel he had a rebuilt family. In one interview without his son, he cried with gratitude and remorse because he no longer felt ashamed of taking his son out in public and also began to enjoy more activities together. In the meantime, the patient's mother, noting her son's improvement in his relationship with his father, began to feel excluded. She shared her jealousies with her therapist. Over several months this led to the ability of both parents to meet together occasionally in the interest of their son. Because father's self-esteem had risen since his regular investment in therapy for himself and his son, he was able to contribute enormously to a new co-parenting relationship with his ex-wife. Their son improved after his parents were able to share and to coordinate their parenthood of him. After the parents had been more successful in coparenting, Mark's day treatment teacher reported a notable increase in Mark's comprehension in reading. He reported that Mark made a lot more sense in class and was less involved in disputes with other children, as well as less chaotic in his impulse control. This illustrates the evolution from parental improvement to classroom behavior and performance. In group therapy, Mark became more outgoing, articulate, and insightful in regard to his own and others' feelings and motivations.

TRANSFERENCE AND COUNTERTRANSFERENCE

Transference

Transference reactions are the unconscious emotions a patient transfers from parents to psychoanalyst, who is seen four times a week, or to a psychodynamic therapist who is seen once or twice a week. Such reactions are what can be termed *new editions with significant new people of old relationships established in infancy or childhood.* This was one of Freud's most insightful discoveries (1910).

In a day treatment center, the psychotherapist who sees the child on a regular and extended basis sooner or later experiences the child's intense and focused transference reactions, which usually can be expressed when the basic real therapeutic relationship becomes stronger and more trustworthy.

Teacher and teaching assistants also become the object of strong transference reactions. However, there are several reasons why such reactions toward the teaching staff are usually more diffuse and less obvious. The child has greater numbers of teaching staff toward whom to express such feelings, and each teacher has a different personality. Teachers usually have professional training that only minimally recognizes such phenomena as transferences. Each teacher often knows less about the individual child's family background and history. Often, children may unconsciously divide or split their transference reactions, attacking a teacher, making extraordinary dependency demands or perhaps sexual gestures toward an assistant teacher, while they are cautiously building up to an intense transference reaction over time to their individual therapist. At home they may be fearfully compliant. Individual psychodynamic child therapists have been trained to look for, and, in a timely and tactful manner, clarify or interpret the child's transference reactions through verbal or metaphoric fantasy or the play activity methods of child psychotherapy.

Countertransference

The Child. Countertransference is the therapist's own unconscious reactions toward the patient or toward the patient's transference, based on unconscious attitudes the individual therapist brings from the therapist's own background (Freud, 1910). Tyson and Tyson (1986) and Schowalter (1986) have reminded child psychiatrists of these phenomena. Schowalter describes countertransference as a currently neglected concept in child psychiatry. He notes that other psychodynamic concepts have also dropped out of the vocabulary and awareness of child psychiatrists. He attributes much of the neglect of countertransference to the current emphasis on descriptive and biological psychiatry. Because it cannot be precisely measured, it has dropped out of favor. Schowalter also reminds us that we have always had powerful unconscious resistance to the serious self-examination required for the recognition of strong countertransference in oneself. He gives examples of how these emotions can be explored in the supervision of child psychiatry trainees. Extreme anger, hate, or fear toward a child are most likely to be noticed because they cause the most anxiety in staff members. It is very painful to admit to having strong, unwarranted, negative reactions toward children. Child patients interact with adult professionals far more motorically and physically than do adults, and this is a major factor in evoking strong countertransference reactions. It is easy when one is restraining a defiant child to hold him or her a little too tightly, influenced by feelings of impatience or hostility.

The Child's Mother. Beiser (1971) observed that those who choose to specialize in work with children often identify with the mother's role and compete to be a better mother. Such therapists may have negative attitudes toward the parents they treat. A balanced viewpoint between children and parents is hard to achieve, but it is vital in child and parent therapy.

Transference and Countertransference among Staff

If transference and countertransference emotions are easy to neglect and hard to work with among clinicians who have often been trained and supervised intensively around these experiences, concern must be expressed about the help special education teachers received around similar issues. In some cases, the basic concepts of transference–countertransference have rarely been discussed and barely understood. How do assistant teachers with less training learn to cope with sudden, extreme, irrational demands, whether sexual, dependent, or hostile, by the children in their care?

The teaching staff as a whole works with children in a day treatment center in classes of six or seven for long periods of time. It is the task of supervisors of teachers to help them with both the concepts and personal experiences of such irrational emotions. Close working relationships, frequent staff rounds, and interdisciplinary seminars can be of immense value. A specific family treatment team must be supportive of each member in dealing with a difficult or divisive child or parent. Disturbed children and their distressed families make intense demands on the staff of a day treatment program.

There are several problems, some of which are administrative. For example, when special educators are officially supervised and paid by city and county special education sections, they may resent supervision by center clinical personnel. The teachers have sometimes been trained to use psychoeducation or psychodynamic understanding as defined by Blom (1979), Long, Morse, and Newman (1980), and Knoblock (1983). Most of the recent emphasis has been on the training of teachers in the use of behavior modification techniques. Thus there may be conflicts around theoretical and clinical approaches between educational and clinical staff members. Integration of dynamic and behavioral approaches by administrators is possible but quite difficult. These issues are likely to give rise to interprofessional transferences and countertransferences. Both teachers and clinicians are among the professions most likely to stimulate transference attitudes from parents as well as children. These several basic conflicts stimulate a number of abrasive interactions between clinicians and special educators. Staff development, conceptual sharing, and collaboration are vitally necessary.

SPECIFIC DYNAMIC SIGNIFICANCE OF DAY TREATMENT

Day treatment is of psychodynamic importance in its own right. It is uniquely adapted to the child's average expectable daytime experiences. It overlaps a child's usual school life, and there are less painful and complex separation anxieties such as those involved in hospitalization or residential treatment. In day treatment the child feels less different and much more of a regular child. In addition, parents, family, and home environment will have been closely evaluated in regard to their basic potential capacities to help their child and achieve parenting stability. They will also have agreed to participate in once-a-week parental or family therapy.

From a medical perspective, day hospital also fits in with Hippocrates's principle of *Primum non nocere* (first, do no harm). Educationally, day treatment reflects current school legislation of the least restrictive alternative.

The uses of time are vital to psychodynamic day treatment. We have never seen it mentioned that day treatment as a total program of 6 to 8 hours a day also has a therapeutic frequency of 5 days a week.

The child's individual psychodynamic therapy does not occupy more than 1 or 2 sessions a week. But the child also has group therapy and is exposed to the complex array of therapeutic educational activities of the school program.

Time-structured programs are vital to all children. The times allotted to cognitive work in class, to expressive exercises such as physical education, music, and art therapy, demand more controlled expressivity than, for example, group therapy. Individual therapy is the freest place of all. A child in such a program learns and experiences tolerance for flexibility and gradients of direction, sternness, moderate supportive expression and relatively free expression. These gradients in relation to specifically different staff relationships can be internalized to strengthen the child's ego. As an example, many borderline children in our program can control much of their pathology and gain increasing normalization because of their internalization of integrated interpersonal relationships, well-defined spaces, and consistent time structure in their therapeutic environment.

Day treatment introduces a number of new adults with special understandings into the child's life and a number of disturbed, disturbing, and improving peers with whom to share recovery. It is the hope of those who participate in the life of a child and his or her family that they will offer increasing tolerance and skillful management of reality, more trusting and gratifying relationships, greater flexibility and expression in play, and richer verbal skills in both cognition and emotional vocabulary.

Emotions such as grief pertain to past losses, whereas guilt and remorse pertain to past wrongdoings. Anxiety is anticipatory. Ego functions in their most mature forms use anticipation constructively to plan for the future. Reality testing, impulse control, and delay of gratification make possible actions that will result in pleasurable creations or events in the future.

The wonderful title, "The Other 23 Hours" (Trieshman, Whittaker, & Brendtro, 1969), concerned itself with what a 23-hour milieu can offer outside the highly esteemed individual therapeutic hours. In day treatment, there are perhaps 16 hours of life each day that are far less understandable, or less understood. Even the most cooperative parents are defensive or unaware of some aspects of the family as a physical and emotional environment. It is a major goal of the therapeutic engagement of parents to build such a trusting relationship that the heavily guarded *past family history* and *past family life* can gradually unfold and be shared, so that the child's other 16 hours might also be susceptible to remediation.

The knowledge that parents are in therapy has a deep impact on the child. The relationship to the institution as a whole is very profound. The setting may be perceived as a power temporarily above the parents. The entire family has a global transference to the institution. As one child said with amazement: "You got doctors here, you got teachers here, and there's no whuppin's." The totality, frequency, and intensity of a day treatment program shares many qualities with psychoanalysis. The regularity and consistency of the time, the place, the program, the staff, and the rituals of coming and going are similar. The program offers places and people where a child can let it "all hang out" and other places where he can be helped to "get it together" to study, to make friends, to paint, to sing, to verbalize his fears and depressions, even to learn words that express joy and happiness.

Many of our children have single parents, and quite a few experience latchkey solitude and anxiety. Many keep secrets about having been beaten, and more than a few have been sexually abused. For some, what they have to report (or conceal) is not a nightmare, but a nightmarish home reality, where parents yell and fight, get divorces, get intoxicated, have new adult relationships, many of which perplex, overstimulate, tease, frighten, or seduce the child who often is desperate for a new parent.

In a day hospital, it is the *night residue* in the child's mind that accompanies the child to school each day. The bad dream may be only one of several painful experiences during each 16 hours to the next. Day treatment provides, for many children, an effective and dynamically significant alternative to intensive residential treatment. The diurnal rhythmicity and bright metaphor of daylight represents the enlightenment of the child and the family.

CONCLUSION

Whether a day treatment program is psychodynamic in an explicit way is not necessarily of primary importance. The unconscious is ubiquitous, psychodynamics are everywhere, and emotions are always present. When a society looks at its families and children with concern, awareness, and a sense of preciousness, there is hope. Unconsciously, a society will create the child and family programs it really needs. Psychodynamic day treatment programs that demonstrate good outcome, such as in those studied by Blom, Farley, and Ekanger (1973) and Zimet, Farley, Silver, Hebert, Robb, Ekanger, and Smith

(1980), indicate a credibility and trustworthiness that deserve and require a high priority in a sensitive and progressive society.

REFERENCES

Abelin, E. L. (1971). The role of the father in the separation-individuation process. In S. McDevitt & C. Settlage (Eds.), *Separation-individuation: Essays in honor of Margaret S. Mahler* (pp. 229–252). New York: International Universities Press.

American Psychiatric Association. (1975). *A psychiatric glossary: The meaning of terms frequently used in psychiatry* (4th ed.). Washington, DC.

Anthony, E. J. (1956). The significance of Jean Piaget for child psychiatry. *British Journal of Medical Psychology, 30,* 20–34.

Anthony, E. J. (1957). The system makers; Piaget and Freud. *British Journal of Medical Psychology, 30,* 255–269.

Anthony, E. J. (1970). The reactions of parents to the oedipal child. In E. J. Anthony & T. Benedek (Eds.), *Parenthood: Its psychology and psychopathology* (pp. 275–288). Boston: Little, Brown & Co.

Beiser, H. R. (1971). Personality characteristics of child analysts: A comparative study of child analyst students and other students as analysts of adults. *Journal of the American Psychoanalytic Association, 19,* 654–669.

Berlin, I. N., & Szurek, S. A. (Eds.). (1965). *Learning and its disorders.* Palo Alto, CA: Science and Behavior Books.

Bernstein, A. E., & Warner, G. M. (1981). *An introduction to contemporary psychoanalysis.* New York: Jason Aronson.

Bettelheim, B. (1950). *Love is not enough: The treatment of emotionally disturbed children.* Glencoe, IL: Free Press.

Bettelheim, B. (1982, March 1). Reflections: Freud and the soul. *The New Yorker,* pp. 52–93.

Bettelheim, B., & Sylvester, E. (1948). The therapeutic milieu. *American Journal of Orthopsychiatry, 18,* 191–206.

Bettelheim, B., & Zelan, K. (1982). *On learning to read: The child's fascination with meaning.* New York: Alfred A. Knopf.

Blom, G. (1979). Psychoeducation in the clinical setting. In J. Noshpitz & S. I. Harrison (Eds.), *Basic handbook of child psychiatry: Therapeutic Interventions, Vol. 3* (pp. 314–333). New York: Basic Books.

Blom, G. E., Farley, G. K., & Ekanger, C. (1973). A psychoeducational treatment program: Its characteristics and results. In G. E. Blom & G. K. Farley (Eds.), *Report on activities of the Day Care Center of the University of Colorado Medical Center to the Commonwealth Foundation.* Denver: University of Colorado Medical Center.

Bowlby, J. (1969). *Attachment & Loss, Vol. 1: Attachment.* London: Hogarth Press.

Brenner, C. (1955). *An elementary textbook of psychoanalysis.* New York: International Universities Press.

Cath, S. H., Gurwitt, A. R., & Ross, J. M. (Eds.). (1982). *Father and child: Developmental and clinical perspectives.* Boston: Little, Brown & Co.

Eagle, M. N. (1984). *Recent developments in psychoanalysis: A critical evaluation.* New York: McGraw-Hill.

Erikson, E. H. (1959). Identity and the life cycle. *Psychological Issues, 1,* 1–171. New York: International Universities Press.

Fraiberg, S. (1969). Libidinal object constancy and mental representations. *The Psychoanalytic Study of the Child, 24*, 9–47.

Freud, A. (1936). *The ego and the mechanisms of defense.* New York: International Universities Press, 1946.

Freud, A. (1926). *The psychoanalytical treatment of children.* New York: International Universities Press, 1951.

Freud, A. (1965). *Normality and pathology in childhood: Assessments in development.* New York: International Universities Press.

Freud, S. (1893–1895). *Studies on hysteria. Standard Edition, Vol. 2.* London: Hogarth, 1955.

Freud, S. (1900). *The interpretation of dreams. Standard Edition, Vols. 4 & 5.* London: Hogarth, 1953.

Freud, S. (1901). *The psychopathology of everyday life. Standard Edition, Vol. 6.* London: Hogarth, 1960.

Freud, S. (1905a). *Three essays on the theory of sexuality. Standard Edition, Vol. 7.* London: Hogarth, 1953.

Freud, S. (1905b). *Jokes and their relation to the unconscious. Standard Edition, Vol. 8.* London: Hogarth, 1960.

Freud, S. (1910). *The future prospects of psychoanalytic theory. Standard Edition, Vol. 11.* London: Hogarth, 1960.

Freud, S. (1923). *The ego and the id. Standard Edition, Vol. 19.* London: Hogarth, 1961.

Greenspan, S. I. (1982). "The second other": The role of the father in early personality formation and the dyadic-phallic phase of development. In S. H. Cath, A. R. Gurwitt, & J. M. Ross, (Eds.), *Father and child: Developmental and clinical perspectives* (pp. 123–138). Boston: Little, Brown & Co.

Harlow, H. F. (1958). The nature of love. *American Psychologist, 13*, 673–685.

Hartmann, H. (1939). *Ego psychology and the problem of adaptation.* New York: International Universities Press, 1958.

Hartmann, H. (1956). The development of the ego concept in Freud's work. *International Journal of Psychoanalysis, 37*, 425–438.

Hartmann, H., Kris, E., & Loewenstein, R. M. (1946). Comments on the formation of psychic structure. *Psychoanalytic Study of the Child, 2*, 11–38.

Herzog, J. M. (1980). Sleep disturbance and father hunger in 18 to 28-month-old boys: The Erlkonig syndrome. *The Psychoanalytic Study of the Child, 35*, 219–233.

Herzog, J. M. (1984). Fathers and young children: Fathering daughters and fathering sons. In J. D. Call, E. Galenson, & R. L. Tyson (Eds.), *Frontiers of Infant Psychiatry, 2*, 335–342. New York: Basic Books.

Hirschberg, J. C. (1953). The role of education in the treatment of emotionally disturbed children through planned ego development. *American Journal of Orthopsychiatry, 23*, 684–690.

Jacobson, E. (1954). The self and the object world: Vicissitudes of their infantile cathexes and their influence on ideation and affective development. *The Psychoanalytic Study of the Child, 9*, 75–127.

Klein, G. S. (1976). *Psychoanalytic theory: An exploration of essentials.* New York: International Universities Press.

Knoblock, P. (1983). *Teaching emotionally disturbed children.* Boston: Houghton Mifflin Co.

Krug, O. (1952). The application of principles of child psychotherapy in residential treatment. *American Journal of Psychiatry, 108*, 695–700.

Long, N. J., Morse, W. C., & Newman, R. G. (1980). *Conflict in the classroom: The education of emotionally disturbed children.* Belmont, CA: Wadsworth.

Mahler, M., Pine, F., & Bergman, A. (1975). *The psychological birth of the human infant: Symbiosis and individuation.* New York: Basic Books.

Newman, C. J., Dember, C. F., & Krug, O. (1973). He can but he won't: A psychodynamic study of so-called "gifted underachievers." *The Psychoanalytic Study of the Child, 28,* 83–129. New Haven: Yale University Press.

Pearson, G. H. J. (1954). *Psychoanalysis and the education of the child.* New York: Norton.

Piaget, J. (1936). *The origins of intelligence in children* (2nd ed.). New York: International Universities Press.

Redl, F., & Wineman, D. (1957). *The aggressive child.* Glencoe, IL: The Free Press.

Roiphe, H., & Galenson, E. (1981). *Infantile origins of sexual identity.* New York: International Universities Press.

Rosen, V. W. (1955). Strephosymbolia: An intrasystemic disturbance of the synthetic function of the ego. *The Psychoanalytic Study of the Child, 10,* 83–99.

Sarnoff, C. (1976). *Latency.* New York: Jason Aronson.

Schowalter, J. E. (1986). Countertransference in work with children: Review of a neglected concept. *Journal of Child Psychiatry, 25,* 40–45.

Shapiro, T., & Perry, R. (1976). Latency revisited: The age 7 plus or minus 1. *The Psychoanalytic Study of the Child, 31,* 79–105.

Solnit, A., & Neubauer, P. (1986). Object constancy and early triadic relationships. *Journal of Child Psychiatry, 25,* 23–29.

Spitz, R. (1945). Hospitalism: An inquiry into the genesis of psychiatric conditions in early childhood. *The Psychoanalytic Study of the Child, 1,* 53–74.

Spitz, R. (1946). Anaclitic depression: An inquiry into the genesis of psychiatric conditions in early childhood. *The Psychoanalytic Study of the Child, 2,* 313–342.

Spitz, R. A., & Cobliner, W. G. (1965). *The first year of life.* New York: International Universities Press.

Sullivan, H. S. (1947). *Conceptions of modern psychiatry.* New York: W. W. Norton.

Sullivan, H. S. (1953). *The interpersonal theory of psychiatry.* New York: W. W. Norton.

Szurek, S. A., Berlin, I. N., & Boatman, M. J. (Eds.). (1971). *Inpatient care for the psychotic child. Vol. 5.* Palo Alto, CA: Science and Behavior Books.

Trieshman, A. E., Whittaker, J. K., & Brendtro, L. K. (1969). *The other 23 hours: Child care work with emotionally disturbed children in a therapeutic milieu.* Chicago: Aldine.

Tyson, R. L., & Tyson, P. (1986). The concept of transference in child psychoanalysis. *Journal of Child Psychiatry, 25,* 30–39.

Westman, J. C. (1979). Psychiatric day treatment. In J. D. Noshpitz & S. I. Harrison (Eds.), *Basic handbook of child psychiatry: Therapeutic interventions, Vol. 3* (pp. 288–299). New York: Basic Books.

Winnicott, D. W. (1952). Anxiety associated with insecurity. *Collected papers: Through pediatrics to psychoanalysis* (pp. 97–100). New York: Basic Books.

Winnicott, D. W. (1953). Transitional objects and transitional phenomena: A study of the first not-me possession. *The International Journal of Psychoanalysis, 34,* 89–97.

Winnicott, D. W. (1965). *The maturational processes and the facilitating environment.* New York: International Universities Press.

Zimet, S. G., Farley, G. K., Silver, J., Hebert, F. B., Robb, E. D., Ekanger, C., & Smith, D. (1980). Behavior and personality changes in emotionally disturbed children enrolled in a psychoeducational day treatment center. *Journal of the American Academy of Child Psychiatry, 19,* 240–256.

8

Day Treatment for Disturbed Children from Socially and Economically Disadvantaged Homes

STEWART GABEL, MARK FINN,
and ROBERT CATENACCIO

INTRODUCTION

The Children's Day Hospital (CDH) of the New York Hospital–Cornell Medical Center, Westchester Division, is a hospital-based day treatment program that has been in existence for about 15 years. It currently serves almost exclusively severely disturbed minority children from urban areas. These children come from economically disadvantaged homes. About 75% of the children are black; most of the rest are white; a few are Hispanic. As will be described more fully, the children at the CDH have a variety of psychiatric diagnoses. The majority have been referred from local school divisions because of conduct problems, impulsivity, and hyperactivity that have made functioning in the local school environment impossible even when

STEWART GABEL • Department of Psychiatry, Cornell University Medical College, New York Hospital–Cornell Medical Center, Westchester Division, White Plains, New York 10605. MARK FINN • Psychology Department, North Central Bronx Hospital, 342 Kossuth Avenue, Bronx, New York 10454. ROBERT CATENACCIO • 512 Mamaroneck Avenue, White Plains, New York 10605.

special services have been provided. Problem areas in the families of these children often include poverty, alcohol or drug abuse, antisocial behavior, and child abuse or neglect. Many of the children live in foster care or with the extended family rather than biological parents. Others live with only one biological parent, almost invariably the mother. No child currently enrolled in the program lives with both biological parents. Social service agency involvement is extremely common.

This chapter will focus on specific aspects of the mental health assessment and treatment of this population. It will emphasize what the CDH has done in the recent past to evaluate the behavioral and emotional characteristics of this population and to develop programs that address problem areas from a mental health standpoint. We will not discuss issues related to providing mental health services to particular minority groups but will focus more broadly on serving a heterogeneous economically disadvantaged population. It should be emphasized, however, that specific mental health programs must be formulated with an awareness of the needs of specific populations who are being served. To be most effective, program design and clinical intervention must be responsive to the personal, familial, social, and cultural characteristics of the population being treated.

The chapter will have five parts. The first part will describe the program in more detail. The second and third parts will discuss diagnostic characteristics of these children and describe our work aimed at developing a broader assessment battery for them and for their families. The fourth part describes the results of a study to evaluate the outcome of these children at the CDH over the last several years. The fifth part describes treatment planning and approaches that are being instituted to help deal with the problems of this group of children and their families.

It should be emphasized that our approach to program planning and evaluation at the CDH is based not only on clinical judgment, although this is obviously crucial, but also on obtaining systematic data for program evaluation and future research efforts. It has been our belief that programmatic strength depends on clinical ability as well as on carefully gathered and analyzed systematic observation.

PROGRAM CHARACTERISTICS

The CDH of the New York Hospital–Cornell Medical Center, Westchester Division, is a multidisciplinary day treatment program for children between the ages of 5 and 12 years who have severe, chronic, behavioral and emotional disorders that cannot be treated adequately by usual outpatient methods and that do not require long-term residential or inpatient care. Nearly all of the children have associated severe family dysfunction. Most have specific learning disabilities in the context of generally normal overall intellectual functioning.

The children in the CDH differ from children admitted to the child inpatient psychiatry unit at New York Hospital–Cornell Medical Center, Westchester Division, in a number of ways. These include their greater degree of social and economic disadvantage, higher rates of reported child abuse/maltreatment, and lower rates of recent suicidal ideation/behavior.

The staff of the CDH consists of a full-time unit chief (a child psychiatrist), one full-time nursing care coordinator, one full-time Master's-level staff nurse, two full-time Master's-level social workers, a half-time PhD staff psychologist, one full-time activities therapist, and four full-time mental health workers. Trainees (two social work, three psychology predoctoral, and one half-time child psychiatry fellow) complete the staffing and serve actively in clinical roles.

The professional clinical and educational staff of the CDH is mainly white, although leadership roles (e.g., unit chief, nursing care coordinator, school principal) have been held by Black staff members. Mental health workers (case aides) and teacher aides have been mainly black, with some individuals in these positions being white.

The program had traditionally emphasized psychodynamic treatment approaches, although, as discussed in the final section, an eclectic approach is now employed. All patients receive individual psychotherapy on a weekly basis, group therapy three times per week, various activity-oriented social skills groups, milieu management, and expressive play experiences on a regular basis. Parent/family contact is encouraged and maintained as much as possible in the face of severe family disorganization. Child-centered parental support and guidance is provided as indicated and feasible.

Throughout the usual 1- to 3-year enrollment of children in the CDH, the youngsters receive educational services through an on-grounds school program run by the White Plains, New York, public schools, under contract with New York Hospital. Three teachers, four teacher aides or assistants, and a secretary and a principal are involved with the school. Most referrals come from school districts in Westchester County after intervention approaches in the local schools have been unable to benefit or control the psychiatric disturbances of these youngsters. Other referral sources such as hospital inpatient units are also important (e.g., Child Inpatient Unit, New York Hospital–Cornell Medical Center). All of the patients are Medicaid recipients because Medicaid is the primary third party payer at present for psychiatric day treatment for children in New York State. Approximately 10 children per year leave the program, resulting in a nearly complete program turnover every 2 to 3 years or so. The enrollment has recently remained at 25 to 26 patients.

DIAGNOSTIC CHARACTERISTICS AND STANDARDIZED ASSESSMENT OF CHILDREN IN THE CDH

Table 1 lists the primary psychiatric diagnoses of children recently enrolled in the CDH, excluding Axis II learning disorders. Diagnoses are based on criteria of the Diagnostic and Statistical Man-

Table 1. Diagnoses of 25 Children in the CDH According to DSM-III Criteria

Axis I	
Conduct disorder, socialized, nonaggressive	2
Conduct disorder, undersocialized, aggressive	6
Conduct disorder, socialized, aggressive	1
Conduct disorder, undersocialized, nonaggressive	1
Attention deficit disorder with hyperactivity	7
Oppositional disorder	4
Dysthymic disorder	3
Elective mutism	1
Mild mental retardation with associated behavioral problems	2
Atypical psychosis	2
Atypical anxiety disorder	1
Infantile autism	1
Separation anxiety disorder	1
Atypical paraphilia	1
Axis II	
Borderline personality disorder	3
Schizotypal personality disorder	1
Histrionic personality disorder	2
Mixed personality disorder with paranoid and aggressive features	1
Mixed personality disorder with dependent and immature features	1
Mixed personality disorder with schizotypal and immature features	1
(Nearly all of the children have severe learning disorders that are not listed here.)	

ual of Mental Disorders, third edition (DSM-III), of the American Psychiatric Association (1980). Diagnoses were obtained by mutually agreed-upon ratings of two of the authors who are child psychiatrists (S. G. and R. C.). (R. C. was, at the time of the ratings, a general psychiatrist completing his child psychiatry fellowship in the CDH.) It is clear that conduct disorder, attention deficit disorder, and oppositional disorder are frequent in this population, as are multiple diagnoses. The rather common occurrence of personality disorder diagnoses indicates that several of these children have long-standing problems of a chronic nature. These children often regress to quite early developmental levels, have significant self-injurious and suicidal tendencies, tend to idealize or denigrate caregivers, and have impulsive tendencies and poor adaptive capacities. Several of these features are characteristic of the borderline personality disorder diagnosis of DSM-III. We make no statement as to whether children with this diagnosis, about which there is much controversy in adult and in child psychiatry, are similar to adults with the disorder of the same name described in DSM-III. We wish to emphasize only that several children in this population of severely disturbed youngsters conform to personality disorder diagnoses in DSM-III.

EFFORTS TOWARD A STANDARDIZED ASSESSMENT

Assessment and treatment of this population present several interrelated and interacting problems related to the children's severe behavioral and emotional disorders: (a) the economic and social disadvantage of the family and (b) family turmoil. Both are a part of their everyday lives.

Traditionally, all children admitted to the CDH have been assessed by several of the various professionals at the CDH (e.g., psychiatry, social work, psychology, education, nursing), according to the usual assessment procedures of that discipline. We believe that additional, more standardized assessments of behavioral functioning in, for example, social, adaptive, and family areas might be helpful for clinical work, program evaluation, and research endeavors.

Choosing and implementing an appropriate assessment battery for these children and their families has proved difficult. Initially, we had planned an assessment battery that included the following measures:

1. *The Piers-Harris Children's Self-Concept Scale (Piers & Harris, 1984).* This measure is generally held to be the best standard measure

of children's self-esteem currently available (Epstein, 1985). Recent reports indicate that it is not overly subject to social desirability response bias that has limited the usefulness of other self-esteem inventories. It has recently been formulated for use with minority and special education groups.

2. *The children's version of the Schedule for Affective Disorders and Schizophrenia, the K-SADS (Puig-Antich, Chambers, & Tabrizi, 1983; Orvaschel, 1985).* This widely used measure was to be administered to each child and parent at the time of admission to establish diagnosis by a standardized method. The procedure requires two separate, approximately 1-hour interviews with parent and child, yielding a DSM-III diagnosis.

3. *The Conners original 39-item Teacher Rating Scale (Conners, 1969, 1973) (see later discussion).*

4. *The Child Behavior Checklist (CBCL) (Achenbach & Edelbrock, 1983).* These latter two scales have been well studied in clinical and research settings and have become standards for evaluating children's behavior by teacher and parent report respectively. The Conners scale has been adopted by the National Institute of Mental Health as part of its standardized assessment for studies of childhood psychopharmacology. The CBCL has the advantage of having scales of social competence as well as behavioral scales to assess psychopathology.

5. *The McMaster Family Assessment Device (FAD) (Epstein, Baldwin, & Bishop, 1983).* The FAD is a 53-item scale yielding seven clinically relevant factors of family functioning including an overall score of general functioning. It has been able to significantly discriminate between clinical and nonclinical populations.

6. *The SCL-90-R (Derogatis, Rickels, & Rock, 1976; Payne, 1985).* The SCL-90-R is a relatively brief, easily understood, self-report instrument for adult psychiatric symptoms and has excellent psychometric properties. We use it to assess parental psychopathology. High scores on the SCL-90-R have been found to correlate with a wide range of other psychiatric measures, ratings, and evaluations (Payne, 1985).

Several of these tests were selected after consultation with Sara Zimet of the Day Care Center, University of Colorado Health Sciences Center. (Personal communication with M. F., April 1986.) (For a description of this data base, please see the chapter by Zimet, Farley, and Avitable in Volume 1.) Lack of personnel to implement all of these rating forms proved to be a problem. A second problem occurred after we had worked to ease the burden of assessment with our limited staff time and had streamlined the battery to include only the

CBCL, the Conners Teacher Rating Form, the Piers-Harris Self-Concept Scale, the SCL-90-R, and the FAD. Parents were often resistant to filling out parent rating forms dealing with their own possible psychopathology (the SCL-90-R) or with family dysfunction (the FAD). Having the Conners Teacher Rating Form and the Piers-Harris Self-Concept Scale completed by teachers and children, respectively (the latter with staff assistance), presented no difficulty. Parental completion of the CBCL was intermediate in difficulty. Parents were often resistant to any outside agency involvement in their lives and seemed to often view requests of the staff for program involvement as intrusive and unwarranted.

In addition, several children lived with relatively short-term foster parents or in other relatively temporary homes with adult relatives whose own possible psychopathology or family dysfunction, as assessed on the SCL-90-R or FAD, might be of limited use in providing long-term care or planning for the child. In short, the shifting nature and instability of these children's lives and homes made even completing assessment forms difficult.

Nevertheless, we persisted with the preceding assessment battery and obtained teacher and self-concept ratings on all the children and parental information for about one-half of the parents or caretakers. The assessments were then scored. As seen in Table 2, the results indicated that all of the children viewed themselves as having either

Table 2. Assessment Battery Results in the CDH

	Percentage of subscales in normal range	Percentage of subscales in deviant range
Piers-Harris Self-Concept Scale (low self-esteem = $T < 40$)	85	15
Conner Teacher Rating Scale (deviant rating = $T > 70$)	57	43
Achenbach Child Behavior Checklist (deviant rating = $T > 70$)	84	16
SCL-90-Revised (deviant rating = $T > 60$)	90	10
Family Assessment Device (deviant rating = scale score > 3)	95	5

average or above average self-esteem as measured by the total score on the Piers-Harris Self-Concept Scale. On the individual subtests of the scale, the children rated themselves as having low self-esteem in only 24 of 156, or 15% of the cases.

The teacher reports, however, as reflected on the Conners Teacher Rating Scale, showed numerous severe problem areas in many of the children tested. The parents' reports of the children's behavior as assessed by the Achenbach Child Behavior Checklist tended to show some problem areas but were closer overall to the children's own assessment of their problems (or lack of problems) than to the teacher assessments. Relatively little psychological or family deviance was shown by parent report on either the SCL-90-R or on the FAD. These results also are summarized in Table 2.

Most of these results contrasted markedly with our clinical assessment of these children who, along with their families, were felt to have severe psychopathology. We interpreted the children's and parents' assessments to reflect either a general lack of trust in the mental health staff or a strong sense of denial about personal and family problems. The children had been assisted in completing the Piers-Harris Self-Concept Scale by mental health workers. These workers function as case aides and often have lived in the same neighborhoods as the children and have known the children for months or years. Because of the children's identification with these case aides who helped them to complete the forms, we felt that distrust of professional staff alone was not an adequate explanation for the children rating themselves as having so few problems with self-esteem. The likelihood of denial of problems by parents and caretakers rather than simple mistrust of staff also seemed probable on clinical grounds and had to be taken into account in further attempts at assessment.

As will be discussed more fully in the final section, we decided to eliminate the SCL-90-R and FAD from our assessment battery because these met with so much resistance and added little useful information regarding our population. For the battery, we decided to substitute therapist ratings of the child's behavior, thereby providing another perspective for all children (Zimet & Farley, 1986). In this way we felt we would have several views of the problem areas of these children. We determined that we would have to place greater weight on professional assessment of problems and changes than might be done in settings in which parents were more cooperative with mental health providers and parental ratings were held to be more valid. This seemed regrettable in part, but also appropriate, because recommendations for these children's future placements and treatment from educational and psychotherapeutic points of view would depend to a considerable degree on professional and teacher assessment and not only on their own or their parents' or caretakers' views of their behavior.

Another issue, of course, became how to address the parents' or caretakers' denial of problems in themselves and their children in the home environment and what this meant programmatically and therapeutically. This will also be discussed in the final section.

OUTCOME OF CHILDREN IN THE CDH

Program planning depends partly on a knowledge of how patients have fared in treatment. With this in mind, Gabel, Finn, and Ahmad (1988) undertook a study to evaluate outcome of children treated in the CDH over the 5 years, 1981–1985 inclusive. Demographic information, diagnoses by DSM-III criteria, family status, history of parental substance abuse, suspected child abuse, suicidality, or severe assaultiveness or aggression were obtained on over 50 consecutive discharges by retrospective chart review. Gabel and his coworkers found that certain preadmission variables seemed to predict the outcome of treatment. Whether a child was recommended for continued residence in a home environment on discharge from the CDH or whether the child was recommended for removal from the home to inpatient hospitalization or residential treatment after his or her treatment in the CDH depended on a number of factors. A prior history of suspected child abuse, parental substance abuse, suicidal ideation/behavior, or severe assaultive behavior prior to entry in the CDH predicted at or near statistically significant levels out-of-home placement despite what was often rather lengthy treatment that averaged about 2 years in the CDH.

Because continued home residence is generally a goal of day treatment, this study seemed to suggest that *for the population served by the CDH,* a largely Black minority population from disadvantaged homes, one might be able to predict which children would do well in day treatment and which children would not do well in day treatment based on preadmission factors. The implications of these findings on program planning, admission criteria, and the institution of new emphases in the program are discussed in the following section.

CURRENT PROGRAM DESIGN AND PLANNING
FOR THE FUTURE

Our clinical experience, review of the literature in dealing with children having the mental health problems described here, and the results of our outcome study have all led to ongoing and anticipated programmatic changes. Several of these will be described in this section.

Interventions with Children

We feel that many children with conduct disorder, impulsivity, and attention deficit disorder with hyperactivity are best treated in an individual sense, based on the current literature, by pharmacologic and/or behavioral therapies, sometimes in association with cognitive approaches. Careful diagnosis and our assessment battery have shown these disorders to be extremely common in our population (see Table 1). Medication and behavioral approaches therefore have been increasingly used in the program. A behavioral approach has been instituted in the milieu.

Because so many of our children also have complex and long-standing psychological problems related to internal feelings, reactions, and conflicts and because their relationships with others (parents, peers, society) are so often problematic, many of the children also receive individual psychodynamically oriented therapy as well. Others have more relationship oriented or supportive approaches on an individual basis. The possibility of childhood depression has also been increasingly considered because depression is so often linked with conduct disorder in preadolescents (Puig-Antich, 1982).

The comprehensive treatment of these children clearly challenges the limits of thoughtful eclecticism. It is our experience that both intrapsychic and behavioral interventions are important. Yet, a genuinely effective integration remains elusive. However, because day treatment is fast becoming one of the few comprehensive treatment settings available for long-term intervention, it may be an ideal setting to generate a clinical grammar for authentic multimodal treatments and to evaluate them systematically.

Interventions with Families

The very disturbed nature of these children's families has also been a constant concern. We now require more family involvement than previously, as agreed to by a written contract with parents that is signed prior to admission. This contract outlines the services provided and states the expectations we have for parents of children in the program. Our feeling is that without family involvement our therapy stands little chance of success.

Our clinical experiences and our assessment battery have also indicated that parents of these children appear remarkably "untroubled" or uninvolved with their children's problem areas, as understood by mental health professionals. It has been extremely difficult to elicit their participation in programmatic efforts to provide help to the children. The apparent denial of their children's problems and the children's own denial is extreme. In order for the program to help these children, we feel that parents must develop more realistic views of their own and their children's problem areas and more effective strategies for dealing with personal and family difficulties. They must also gain greater trust in mental-health-care providers. All of this appears to be unlikely without therapeutic contact. The view of some mental health providers that a child should be maintained and served in a therapeutic program in the hope that he or she will benefit, even if the parent does not participate, seems unrealistic for the majority of these children who return to disturbed homes and families each evening.

Actual therapy for this group of parents and families now takes the form of parent guidance and/or behavioral work. We are currently also conducting a parent group in which general parenting issues can be discussed and support given. Home visits are also utilized a great deal for both assessment and ongoing treatment. There are some parents who are reluctant to discuss problems in a clinic or day hospital setting. Some of these same parents are pleased to welcome clinicians who show interest into their homes, where they appear more relaxed, appreciative of the extra effort made for the home visit, and more open to personal discussions. (The topic of home visits is discussed by Ekanger in Volume 1.)

Other Interventions

Our clinical impressions, coupled with our outcome study, have also indicated that parental substance abuse and child abuse/maltreatment are major problems in this group of families. We are now much more active in assessing and actively intervening in these areas with our children and their families. Our contacts with social service agencies have also increased considerably, and we have become even more active in advocating for the child. Surprisingly to some, our active intervention with child protective services and social service departments around issues of child abuse and maltreatment has resulted only in short-term resistance and anger on the part of parents. Greater involvement and alliance with clinical staff has been common in the longer term. We try to give clear, firm, supportive messages to parents that our role includes helping the child to be safe, protected, and nurtured, as well as helping them to help their children toward these ends. We recognize that agency pressure is sometimes necessary to achieve these goals.

Most of the parents in our program have strong desires to keep their children in home residence with them despite what may have been their own maltreatment of the children. Outside agency involvement is often correctly perceived as a threat to remove the child from the home. This sometimes serves as a needed stimulus for the parent to begin working on his or her and the child's problems. Generally, the children, after a short period of anger, fear, and resistance, feel comfortable knowing that their needs are cared for, even if their parents cannot provide for the care themselves and need outside agency "pressure" and assistance.

Assessing Change

As noted earlier, we feel that purely clinical assessment of outcome is inadequate and that it is important to assess changes more systematically over time in the children and families we serve. Our current assessment battery is shorter than we would have hoped because of the problems noted earlier. The battery accepts the limitations of time, funding, and population characteristics. As described earlier, it consists of the Piers-Harris Self-Concept Scale, completed by the child with staff assistance; the CBCL filled out by the parent; the CBCL (parent form) filled out by the therapist; and the Conners Teacher Rating Form filled out by the teacher. All of these are done once a year. It is our feeling that in this multiproblem and therapeutically resistant group of children and parents, numerous views of behavior problems and behavioral changes over time are needed for balanced clinical judgments and recommendations concerning future therapy and education.

Day Treatment for Whom

Finally, our outcome study has indicated to us that particular children do well in our day treatment program and others do not.

Child abuse, parental substance abuse, suicidality, and severe assaultiveness prior to admission have been associated with poor outcome and out-of-home placement recommendations on discharge. We feel it is necessary to consider these factors strongly in our admission evaluation. It is important to realize that day treatment is a useful modality for many children but that it has not been effective in our program for many of the most severely disturbed children who have suicidal ideation, severely assaultive behavior, or who have suffered massive family related disturbances and who have little or no ongoing family support. Our admission evaluations have begun to reflect this assessment and some children, formerly thought acceptable for admission, have now been viewed much more cautiously.

We have, on the other hand, become more therapeutically focused and active in dealing with child abuse, parental substance abuse, suicidal ideation and depression, and severe assaultiveness for those who are accepted into the program. Our hope is that, in focusing on these areas therapeutically, we will allow some children who might not have benefited previously to now benefit from our day treatment program and remain in the home environment.

REFERENCES

Achenbach, T. M., & Edelbrock, C. S. (1983). *Manual for the Child Behavior Checklist and Revised Child Behavior Profile*. Burlington, VT: Author.

American Psychiatric Association (1980). *Diagnostic and statistical manual of mental disorders (3rd ed.)*. Washington, DC: Author.

Conners, C. K. (1969). A teacher rating scale for use in drug studies with children. *American Journal of Psychiatry, 126*, 884–888.

Conners, C. K. (1973). Rating scales for use in drug studies with children. Pharmacotherapy of children [Special issue]. *Psychopharmacology Bulletin, 9*, 24–84.

Derogatis, L. R., Rickels, K., & Rock, A. F. (1976). The SCL-90 and the MMPI: A step in the validation of a new self report scale. *British Journal of Psychiatry, 128*, 280–289.

Epstein, J. H. (1985). Review of the Piers-Harris Children's Self-Concept Scale. In J. V. Mitchell (Ed.), *Ninth mental measurements yearbook* (pp. 1167–1169). Lincoln: Buros Institute of Mental Measurements of the University of Nebraska-Lincoln.

Epstein, N. B., Baldwin, L. M. & Bishop, D. S. (1983). The McMaster Family Assessment Device. *Journal of Marital and Family Therapy, 9*, 171–180.

Gabel, S., Finn, M., & Ahmad, A. (1988). Day treatment outcome with severely disturbed children. *Journal of the American Academy of Child and Adolescent Psychiatry, 27*, 479–482.

Orvaschel, H. (1985). Psychiatric interviews suitable for use in research with children and adolescents. *Psychopharmacology Bulletin, 21*, 737–745.

Payne, R. W. (1985). Review of the SCL-90-R. In J. V. Mitchell (Ed.), *Ninth mental measurements yearbook* (pp. 1326–1329). Lincoln: Buros Institute of Mental Measurements of the University of Nebraska–Lincoln.

Piers, E. V., & Harris, D. B. (1984). *The Piers-Harris Children's Self-Concept Scale: Revised manual.* Los Angeles: Western Psychological Services.

Puig-Antich, J. (1982). Major depression and conduct disorder in prepuberty. *Journal of the American Academy of Child Psychiatry, 21,* 118–128.

Puig-Antich, J., Chambers, W. J., & Tabrizi, M. A. (1983). The Clinical assessment of current depressive episodes in children and adolescents: Interviews with parents and children. In D. P. Cantwell, & G. A. Carlson (Eds.), *Affective disorders in childhood and adolescence: An update* (pp. 157–179). New York: SP Medical and Scientific Books.

Zimet, S. G., & Farley, G. K. (1986). Four perspectives on the competence and self-esteem of emotionally disturbed children beginning day treatment. *Journal of the American Academy of Child Psychiatry, 25,* 76–83.

9

An Afterschool Day Treatment Program

ELLIE F. STERNQUIST

OVERVIEW

The concept of utilizing a day treatment model for children and adolescents represented an extension of adult models whose history dated to the 1930s in Russia (Wirth, 1986). Children's day treatment models were initiated in the late 1930s in America as a result of the growing awareness by mental health providers of the need to implement less restrictive concepts of care for children than were possible in hospital settings (Evangelakis, 1980).

In California, the evolution of day treatment for children and adolescents was a direct response to legislation (California Welfare and Institutions Code, 1979) requiring the counties to create alternatives to hospitalization for adults. The legislative impetus to deinstitutionalize patients and move them to less restrictive levels of care filtered down to the youth population (California Welfare and Institutions Code, 1983). Public services systems also became more sensitive to the need for multiple levels of care for youngsters who might have been hospitalized arbitrarily because of the absence of more appropriate, less intensive forms of care.

Economic factors prompted changes of significance to families. Increasing numbers of dual career households coupled with an ex-

ELLIE F. STERNQUIST • P.O. Box 514, 3419 Harborview Drive, Gig Harbor, Washington 98335.

pansive growth in the numbers of single-parent families led to the identification of the "latchkey kid" syndrome, or youngsters left to fend for themselves after school while parents were at work and unable to provide child care. Many of these children, who might previously have been hospitalized, were not only left unsupervised but were identified as emotionally disturbed as well. This observation more than any other forced this author's attention to the modification of the concept of day treatment to include an after-school-hours treatment component.

Simultaneously, there was increasing public acknowledgment of child abuse and molestation bringing to light an awareness of impact of childhood experience on adult behavior. The public's sense of urgency led to a greater acceptance of, and advocacy for, the funding of treatment for children and adolescents who had been the victims of these abuses. Mental health professionals, influenced by the family therapy movement, as well as public mental health administrators, began to recognize both the value of family treatment and its cost effectiveness as well.

RATIONALE FOR AN AFTER-SCHOOL-HOURS DAY TREATMENT MODEL

The intent of an afterschool day treatment model is to carry the concept of deinstitutionalization to its fullest ramifications. It represents a commitment to maintain a youngster in the school, home, and family setting insofar as each is able to respond to the special needs of the troubled youngster. An after-school-hours program assumes that educators are best equipped to educate, that families are best suited for child rearing, or alternatively, that responsible adults can create familylike settings and that most youngsters will benefit from remaining in their communities while receiving mental health care. Maintenance in the community fosters parent participation, discourages the stigmatization often associated with hospitalization, and virtually eliminates the regression that is often seen upon reentry into the home, school, and community.

An after-school-hours program demands the creation and coordination of cooperative case management style. Other systems are encouraged and supported in taking their respective responsibilities for the well-being of the youngster and family. It further allows mental health professionals to exercise their expertise without replicating the efforts of others with specialization in such fields as education, social service, and juvenile justice. An after-school-hours model fulfills mental health needs while also being highly responsive to the critical gap in child care common to the latchkey kid. The afterschool model also allows significant flexibility in providing specifically therapeutic and psychosocial services to the youth and family because of the relative freedom from the constraints of the educational setting within which most day treatment programs operate.

PROGRAM DEVELOPMENT

The original program model was conceived and developed in 1979–1980 in conjunction with an adolescent outpatient program at Tri-City Mental Health Authority in Pomona, California. Both clinicians and families were frustrated by the continuing difficulties these youngsters showed: their lack of progress in managing day-to-day issues in school and at home and their probable return to, or entry into, hospitals as a result of many treatment failures. Parents appeared exhausted, doubtful of treatment, helpless, and often without further financial resources to support any additional inpatient expenses.

A 4-day-per-week, after-school-hours program was designed to provide group therapy and socialization activities to a maximum of 14 youngsters ages 13 to 17 over the period of a 6-month experimental program. The program, incidentally, was generated and conducted without additional funding. It drew on the grace of agency management and time sharing of staff from the adolescent outpatient unit and the adult day treatment staff.

Of the 14 youngsters referred to the program, 8 had a history of psychiatric hospitalization totaling more than 160 days of inpatient care within the 12 months before beginning outpatient treatment. During the 6-month trial program and for 6 months following its termination, a total of only 8 days of hospitalization was utilized for one youngster. The program clearly demonstrated both the potential for the model and its efficacy in terms of comparisons of cost-effectiveness.

In 1979–1980, community mental health planners had advocated some form of day treatment for children and adolescents within the catchment area of the San Gabriel Valley of Los Angeles County. In Fiscal Year 1980–1981, the Los Angeles County Department of Mental Health allocated $300,000 for an innovative day treatment program for the youth population. Following the mandates of the

Community Residential Treatment System (California Welfare and Institutions Code, 1983), and the state funding requirements, the county sought a strongly psychosocial and community-based day treatment model.

Pacific Clinics (formerly Pasadena Guidance Clinics), anticipating the county's request for proposals, asked me to conduct a community needs assessment. It was clear that the catchment area would benefit from a day treatment program for children and adolescents. At issue was whether potential referral sources would support an after-school-hours model and what steps would need to be taken to create the networking relationships so crucial to the success of such a model.

The needs assessment consisted of interviews with educators, social services workers, probation department staff, clergy, public and private mental health providers, and other providers of youth activities. The results strongly endorsed the need for the after-school-hours model with a preference for its extension into the evening hours and weekend days as well. If only a portion of the time frame could be accommodated, the after-school-hours (from approximately 2 PM–6 PM) were seen as the most critical. The consensus was that all youth were vulnerable in the absence of effective supervision, but clearly the emotionally disturbed youngsters were at an extreme risk because of the absence of both supervision and treatment.

Two predominant concerns emerged from the interviews. All respondents agreed that excellent relationships would have to be developed with each of the 40 school districts in the catchment area and would need to address personnel at all the levels within each district. A second expressed concern was that the program would have to implement an unusually strong affirmative action program to acknowledge the multiple language and cultural needs of the residents of the catchment area.

The needs assessment also indicated that, optimally, the program should respond to the mental health needs of teen school dropouts, abuse and molestation victims, alternative families (nonnuclear, nontraditional), youth before and after psychiatric hospitalization, substance abusers, and gang youth.

In the spring of 1981, the agency's president and I wrote the proposal. It offered services to 24 youth, ages 7–17, and their families, 5 afternoons and 4 evenings per week and included some Saturday activities. In November 1981, a contract for services in the amount of $303,000 was awarded to Pacific Clinics.

PROGRAM PHILOSOPHY

The program philosophy incorporated its original funding mandate to provide services consonant with the legislative requirements of the Community Residential Treatment System (California Welfare and Institutions Code, 1979, 1983). Treatment was to be innovative and was to be provided in a noninstitutionalized setting. The treatment environment, ambience, and applied practices, commonly referred to as the milieu, were designed to encourage socially constructive experiences and to replicate the relationships that typify those usually found in a healthy child–adult environment. The therapeutic focus was placed on interpersonal interactions with adults, peers, and interage (sibling) groups, with an emphasis on facilitating intrapsychic and developmental mastery of age-appropriate skills and personal and social awareness.

The program also was committed to providing as much continuity as possible between other daily systems in the youngster's life by active case management. The theme of systems relationships and cooperation dominated the program. Using the concept of community systems, the program attempted to engage the full scope of daily systems within which the youngster and the family functioned in order for day treatment to achieve its goals.

Believing that change and unpredictability are relative constants in the human environment, the program purposefully incorporated increasing demands on the youngsters to learn and demonstrate developmentally useful skills when confronting environmental changes and human unpredictability. The intent was to enable the youngster to develop understanding, empathy, self-confidence, and self-control in place of confusion, reactivity, and impulsivity.

The program philosophy also extended to the families or adults responsible for the youngster. Their continuing involvement was required if the youngster was to receive care. In the course of treatment, parents were expected to take increasing responsibility for the supervision and daily routines of the youngsters.

PROGRAM ORGANIZATION

The program is organized into four treatment groups or components. Each is roughly defined by age and developmental capability. They are 6- to 8-year-olds; 9- to 11-year-olds; 12- to 14-year-olds; and

15- to 17-year-olds. Each is staffed by three people, at least one of whom is a trained clinician who functions as the component leader/ supervisor. The other two staff members may be either a clinician– trainee and a paraprofessional counselor, or two paraprofessionals, one of whom has more experience.

Youngsters receive a minimum of 1 and a maximum of 4 hours per week of individual therapy. Family treatment, either in session or group, is approximately 1 hour per week. These services are provided by a licensed, or license-eligible clinician, or a clinician–trainee under the supervision of a licensed clinician. The youngsters spend most of their day in the component group or a partial component group. They are taken out of groups for their individual sessions, and as needed, for psychological testing or psychiatric consultations.

The groups assist the youngster in developing age-appropriate skills and provide a peer support group for exposing and resolving their difficulties. The groups use a multimodal approach structured into a daily curriculum to encourage individuality and social success within the context of the peer and adult interaction system.

The daily curriculum begins with a community meeting and snack for each component and ends with a "rap-up" group in each component. As with all groups or activities scheduled in the course of the day, however, the structure and purpose of the groups reflect developmental competencies both of the age group and the specific youngsters within the group at any given time. This is evidenced most dramatically in the group therapies. Each component schedules a minimum of 2 hours a week of group therapy and often more. The older youngsters most often rely on verbal modalities interspersed with appropriate social-learning activities. The younger groups are more likely to use play-therapy models that encourage and support expression and awareness of feelings without demanding systematic verbal and cognitive skills.

Other scheduled activities occur at the same time in order to best use available staff members. These activities vary distinctly in their content even when bearing the same title. Art therapy, recreational therapy, social skills, computer therapy, field trips, cultural identity, and myriad-component specific groups are each developmentally de- signed. Groups are also flexible enough to remain sensitive to the component members and their frequent personal and group crises. When a group nears homogeneity by diagnosis or history, the curricu- lum can target those related issues or can allow for partial-component groups to be created on a short-term basis to focus on specific needs.

Another source of curriculum variation is seasonal. In summer, for example, a day of therapy is exchanged for swimming at a community pool. Holidays are incorporated through the cultural identity groups, and routines are altered to include multicultural holiday celebrations.

Once a month, a Saturday family therapeutic event is planned for all youngsters, their siblings and parents, and staff. When available, tickets to events like baseball games are offered to families to encourage them to interact socially with their youngsters without depending on the program or staff.

PROGRAM SIZE, STAFFING, AND BUDGET

Since its inception in November 1981, the program has grown from an annual budget of $303,000 serving 24 youths ages 7 to 17 to approximately $767,000 serving 43 youths ages 6 to 17 plus an additional 20 in the mini-, or "waiting list" program. Current cost for a unit of service, or 1 day including all related services at the clinic, is $98 per youngster per day.

Staffing is directed toward accomplishing several goals. One goal is to insure a staff to youngster ratio that assures the physical safety and emotional well-being of all. Currently there are 24.3 full-time equivalent staff to 43 enrolled youngsters. The average daily attendance is 33 youths. Hence the average daily staff to youngster ratio is 1:1.4.

The staff is divided approximately equally between the professional and paraprofessional levels. The latter personnel includes component counselors, activities support staff, clerical, and van drivers. The professional staff is comprised of clinical and clinical/administrative staff representing the disciplines of psychology, social work, marriage and family counseling, psychiatry, and art therapy. The program also provides training opportunities for graduate students in art therapy, psychology, and social work.

The staff are ethnically diversified to reflect the community at large. Additionally, efforts are made to maintain a familylike setting by mixing male and female staff both in the component groups and in the staff as a whole.

The role of the clinician is critical in the staffing and treatment systems. Every enrolled youth is under the immediate care of a clinician who is supervised weekly by a licensed professional. The clinician has the final responsibility for the treatment planning, provision of individual and family therapy, and integration of treatment among all sectors of the program and within the staff. The clinician is also responsible for all aspects of case management including coordination with schools, social services systems, and probation departments. A part-time psychiatric consultant sees every youngster upon entry into the program, schedules sessions with those who are medicated, consults with the clinicians and program staff regularly, and provides consultant services to the outside medical/psychiatric community as well.

Maintenance of the program organization and quality is heavily dependent on adequate staffing. Several times in the program's history, the staffing pattern has been adapted to improve quality of service and relieve undue stress on staff as a result of "role diffusion" or doing too many tasks under the heading of one job description. Upward movement of staff has been encouraged, with successful results. Hourly salary rates are competitive with other comparable southern California mental health settings.

On a day-to-day basis, position vacancies, vacation and sick leave absences, and client emergencies drawing staff away from their routine coverage are filled by other staff on a priority of need premise or by temporary employees. The budget allows funds to hire daily or short-term temporary help to respond to staffing needs at any time. The budget also allows for hiring staff trainers as necessary.

PROGRAM MANAGEMENT

A management team system has been used to direct the course of the program. It is comprised of the program director, assistant director, clinical coordinator, and program coordinator. The program director is accountable to the agency President/CEO and top level staff. The composition of the team has been altered many times to adjust to the increased size, budget, and management requirements of the program.

Dangers of a Growing Closed System

Management has consistently been confronted with two factors that have forced consideration of changes and, occasionally, disruptions in the management team style. The first issue is that the program, unlike many others, is essentially a free-standing one. Although part of a corporate mental health structure, the program shares neither space nor staff with any other program within the Pacific Clinics organization. Inevitably, the staff, youngsters, and parents suffer the consequences of becoming a closed community whose perceptions and moods reflect only the field of players at the time. To create and sustain a viable organization and management direction, management has embodied experimental techniques with varying degrees of success. Each change has been accompanied by the creative tension of the change that has sometimes been difficult for staff to absorb.

The second issue influencing management style has been the annual and often substantial growth of the program. The frequency of mandated changes in quality control, from basic record keeping to staffing and supervisory accountability, have taxed the policymaking and enforcement charge of the managers. With revision of internal systems a constant, little energy is left to foster an ambiance supportive of innovative treatment models. In light of both the closed community issue and the growth demands, it has been difficult to achieve a stable and productive management style.

The program director is accountable for all day-to-day operations to the agency president/CEO. Fiscal management, however, occurs at the corporate office. The director and president/CEO generally meet once a week alone and again at the agency administrative management meeting. These meetings foster the coalescence of agency and program goals and maintain peer/collegial contacts with directors of other sites. They also function as the primary conduit of information flow between the agency's management and the program's management and staff.

Internal program management is accomplished by weekly management team meetings and a combination of staff supervision sessions and daily staff meetings. Each staff member has an assigned supervisor, and 1-hour supervision sessions are required weekly. These sessions provide both a quality assurance and a problem-solving mechanism. They also assist in and encourage two-way information flow among all levels of staff. Daily staff meetings strive to meet staff and management needs for dialogue and cohesion regarding significant clinical and programmatic issues that are not the common material of individual supervision sessions. Of no less importance, daily staff meetings allow staff to express frustration, air differences, and generally engage on a more personal basis with each other.

PROGRAM SYSTEMS (ENTRY TO DISCHARGE)

Referrals to the afterschool program most often come from the school districts and public or private mental health providers, including hospitals. In the past 2 years, referrals from the Department of

Social Services have nearly doubled, however, and account for almost 50% of initial referrals. The referral sources include physicians, juvenile probation officers, and word of mouth.

Typically, the referral source contacts the assessment coordinator by telephone and may follow up with written information. If the youngster meets the broad criteria for probable admission, the referral source contacts the parent. The parent then contacts the assessment coordinator to schedule an assessment interview.

The broad criteria for both candidacy and admission to the program are centered around the concept that the program must serve those youngsters most in need of alternatives to institutionalization. The assessment process considers a history of previous outpatient mental health care that has not met the needs of the youngster. It attends to the need for transitional care in a postdischarge situation from either a hospital or out-of-home placement and carefully evaluates the possibilities of the program providing a treatment alternative to either of the aforementioned.

The clinical criteria were established as a result of the recognition of physical control issues related to keeping the site both open and safe, without locked doors, physical restraints, or full-time physician coverage. Hence, by exclusion, youngsters are not accepted who present with histories of habitual violent acting-out behavior, frequent substances abuse (i.e., polydrug abuse or addiction), or arson.

The assessment interview, usually conducted with both the youngster and parent(s) present, follows a semistructured format. It is facilitated by either a clinician or psychiatrist and generally takes about 1½ hours.

Following this interview, the decision-making process begins. Most often, the interviewing clinician presents the case to the clinical director and one other member of the management staff. If there is an opportunity for an immediate admission to a component group versus being placed on the waiting list, the clinician for the appropriate age group is asked to join in the decision making. If there is a lack of consensus, however, the case may be presented at a total staff meeting. Once a decision is reached, the parent(s) and referral source are notified. If the youngster is not to be admitted, attempts are made to locate appropriate treatment facilities, whether more or less restrictive, and often program staff assists the family in connecting with the new facility.

Due to the high demand for services, there is nearly always a waiting list. The delay in actual entry into the 5-day-a-week program averages 7 weeks but can extend to 3 months. For an admission to be completed, there must be both a place open in the component group and a clinician to take the case. Planning for admissions takes into account language needs of the non-English-speaking families and the monolingual-preferent youngsters in terms of assignment to language-matched clinicians. This factor often forces a reevaluation of priority of need for service.

The waiting list often contains as many as 25 youngsters and families. Because of the severity of difficulties these families experience in the absence of treatment, several years ago the program responded by creating a preadmissions "miniprogram." Drawing on existing staff and operating within the overall budget of the program, the miniprogram was designed to assist the youth and families while they were in a holding pattern. We hoped that some therapeutic contact versus none would lower the risks of client decompensation.

The miniprogram offers a program orientation, weekly multifamily group therapy, group therapy for both the latency-aged children and the adolescents, psychiatric and medication consultation as needed, and some availability of crisis intervention and case management. What is not available is individual and family therapy, 5-day-a-week treatment, and transportation. The miniprogram, although far from treatment panacea, has been of dramatic assistance to both the youngsters and their families. It has also assisted staff in expediting treatment strategies because the youngsters are more familiar with the regular program by the time they actually enter it. Although the wait for full admission can be as long as 3 months, the miniprogram averages 7 weeks. It also is observed that among families who have participated in the miniprogram there is a stronger commitment to participation in the full-time program and a concurrent reduced frequency of parent withdrawal of the youngster from treatment prematurely.

Once admitted to the 5-day-a-week program, a clinician becomes responsible for the case. Treatment plans are formulated, and a process of treatment evaluation is initiated. Routine case review is at the 2-week mark and every 4 weeks thereafter and occurs at case conference meetings set for that purpose. Parents, youngsters, teachers, and significant others are not at those meetings; however, their input is generally solicited either in sessions or telephone consultations prior to the case conferences. Youngsters who are experiencing serious difficulties in treatment are placed on the critical list that allows for a weekly rather than monthly case conference.

As soon as the youngster demonstrates progress in the three arenas of home, school, and program, discussion begins regarding discharge planning. Notably, the order in which program improvement is evidenced appears fairly consistent. The youngster first demonstrates behavioral improvement at school, then at home, and lastly, in the program. Although this is trying for staff, the process suggests that the youngsters learn interpersonal and behavioral skills more rapidly than they do the intrapsychic, workingthrough skills that they need to continue to resolve their difficulties. They also appear to gain trust in bringing their problems to the program while containing them in their routine day-to-day functions. It is sometimes challenging for staff to initiate discussion of a discharge when in fact the youngster's behavior in the program is more disturbed than upon entry. It is also occasionally difficult to convince parents to allow the youngster to remain in treatment when all seems improved at home. Outcome data (Wirth, 1986), however, strongly substantiates that this final phase of treatment is crucial to the integration of coping skills.

Discharge planning also includes a process of weaning the youngster and family from intensive treatment. This is done by first contracting with them for a day off from the program, thus reducing their attendance to 4 days a week. The parent and youngster are encouraged to replace the treatment day with an age-appropriate and structured activity such as scouting or a recreational activity. The youngster is closely monitored for a period of 4 to 6 weeks, and, if problems arise, he or she is able to return to the program immediately on a 5-day schedule.

If all goes well, a second day off is planned. The youngster and parent(s) are encouraged to use this as a free but supervised day. The intent is to test the youngster's resourcefulness, self-confidence, and competence to manage in the larger community of siblings, family, peers, and parents. Four weeks are usually allowed for this trial period with the same option existing of returning to the program full time if necessary.

Simultaneously with the introduction of the days-off schedule, parents are advised to initiate contact with an outpatient facility for further treatment. The goal of the termination process is to successfully connect the family with their new provider before the youngster has been graduated from the program. To assist in this process, the clinicians remain available to the family for therapy sessions and case management contacts for 4 weeks following the formal discharge.

The client follow-up system includes telephone contact with the family and the youngster at 6 weeks, 3 months, and 6 months following termination.

PROGRAM CHALLENGES

The primary challenge of an afterschool day treatment program is to achieve a pragmatic integration of treatment and community resources. A failure to accomplish that single task spells the failure of the treatment intervention. Afterschool day treatment cannot be successful if it operates in a social systems vacuum.

Focal in an afterschool program is the maintenance of excellent relations with the educational providers with whom the youngsters have daily or frequent contacts. Regular communication between school and day treatment personnel, although time consuming, is crucial in creating a sense of continuity for the youngster between the two systems. Because the program assumes advocacy responsibility for the youngster and because nearly 50% of program youth appear in need of educational evaluation for placement in the proper class setting, the possibilities of systems conflicts are ever present. To protect cooperative relationships with the schools, our clinicians have developed sophistication in advocacy and mediation as well as an understanding of the resources and constraints available within each school district involved. This role is well beyond the parameters of the training of most clinicians and requires that we train and supervise our staff carefully so as not to alienate significant players in the districts.

Visits to the schools by the clinician to observe the youngster in the classroom or on the playground, to meet and plan behavioral management strategies with teachers, and to participate in creating individualized educational plans go a long way toward maintaining cordial relations. Teachers and other school personnel are also invited to the afterschool program site at least twice during the schoolyear. Many come more frequently to join in crisis resolution, treatment planning, and problem-solving groups. Telephone contact is encouraged, and written information is exchanged regularly. Additionally, the program offers support to the school districts by providing occasional in-service sessions to their staff, by doing second-opinion assessment interviews free of charge from time to time, and by assisting them with referrals when they are requested.

Other systems also must be fully engaged. Nearly 50% of the youngsters served in Fiscal Year 1986–1987 also were on the rolls of the Department of Public Social Services. Approximately 50% of them, or 25% of the program population, were in out-of-home placement concurrent with their day treatment stay. Furthermore, most of those youngsters also were involved with a social worker, legal and court personnel, an advocate or guardian ad litem, outside psychiatric worker, foster family, and, occasionally, their biological family.

Nearly 40% of the youngsters treated have histories of previous psychiatric hospitalization. Many remain involved with outside psychiatrists, physicians, case managers, or placement workers. In all instances, it is imperative that the day treatment clinician integrate these providers and systems into a caring and cooperative treatment network. Implicit in this community systems concept, however, is that the day treatment role is central to the well-being of the youngster, and hence, responsible for the overall care of the youngster. Although most often appreciated by other providers, the level of responsibility assumed by day treatment has sometimes been a source of conflict, competition, systems dominance, and territoriality within other agencies. When such issues arise, a supervisor or member of management staff intercedes to smooth ruffled feathers.

Staff Training and Education

A related challenge is to provide supportive training and education to day treatment staff to accommodate their need for using extensive case management as part of a comprehensive treatment strategy. This challenge has been met by creating a staffing pattern that allows sufficient time for staff members to engage in consultation and case management. Although cost in staff hours may be high, clinician involvement in those functions ensures that the program does not become isolated and that the youngsters will not be treated in a vacuum.

Parent Involvement

One of the more poignant challenges of day treatment is that of securing successful involvement of the parent/responsible adult. The continuing necessity to evaluate if the youngster is safe in his or her home at night demands the full attention of the treatment staff and requires parent participation in the treatment process. A youngster who has manifested emotional or behavioral difficulties during the day requires a supportive family at night and over the weekends. Likewise, a family experiencing the therapeutic dissolution of habitual and nonconstructive behaviors requires and deserves staff support in coping with the unique needs of the youngster returning to the home each evening.

Early on, the program met the challenge of engaging the parents and establishing therapeutic alliances with them. By reframing the idea that they might be resistant to treatment into the concept that they might be overwhelmed by the multiple conflicts that getting treatment generates, efforts were made to anticipate and eliminate as many obstructions as possible. In nearly all admissions histories, the family and youngster have had previous disappointments in treatment. There has been family financial duress, frustration about time commitments, uncertainty and instability in school placement, and an overall distrust of caregivers.

The program offers transportation to and from the site to those youngsters who need it. It fills a gap in child care from after school until the parent arrives at home. Evening child care is provided for siblings when parents come in for treatment. Specialized parent-support groups such as single-parent groups, gay-parent groups, and adoptive-parent groups are provided as the population warrants them.

These offerings are seen as the initial step in building a therapeutic alliance and providing the parents with a new perspective about what might be available to them as a result of participating in day treatment. In fact, many parents report feeling rewarded for their participation.

The diagnostic and treatment planning processes consume considerable effort by the staff members during the youngster's first 2 weeks in the program. Those involved in the diagnostic and treatment planning workup include the assessment clinician, the psychiatrist, the milieu staff members with whom the youngster interacts, the assigned clinician, the supervisor, and the clinical director. Information gathered from outside sources also is included. At the initial case conference, diagnosis is determined, and treatment goals and strategies are recommended. While the diagnostic approach had used the multi-axial structure of DSM-III (1980), the broader effort of the diagnostic team is to define a view of the youngster's intrapsychic and interpersonal "style" in the environment. From this perspective, the treatment plan then becomes a consideration of what can be done to assist the youngster and family in developing more constructive thought processes and social/interaction skills.

The highly diverse ethnic and socioeconomic area serviced has created unusual challenges to all aspects of the program's operation. In response, management has made a firm and enthusiastic commitment to affirmative action. Staffing has always closely replicated the ethnic diversity of the catchment area and, hence, has facilitated communication among the patients and staff. A complication of the replication standard for staffing, however, has been increased levels of staff stress when positions remain open and existing staff or temporary employees must cover the vacancies until the multiple criteria for hiring have been fulfilled.

Another impact on the program has been that the tensions among the ethnic groups in the larger community have been brought into the program. The therapeutic environment was frequently disrupted by the projections of that tension. In 1984, additional funding was secured to initiate a new program, the Cultural Identity program, to resolve therapeutically some of these problems. It was developed with an age-appropriate curriculum for each component, and a clinician was hired to direct the program. The goals included learning to experience pride in oneself and one's heritage without sacrificing understanding and acceptance of the differences of others. This effort has greatly reduced prejudice and stereotyping in both the youngsters and the staff. An indication of the success of this curriculum is that many local schools have requested that it be implemented in their settings. When staff are available, they have participated in introducing such groups at school sites.

The program provides therapeutic services in multiple languages and is committed to offering all services with sensitivity to cultural values. These "gifts," or ethnically and therapeutically sensible aspects of service provision (Sue, 1986), appear to substantially increase parent involvement and support positive treatment outcomes. This brings about further continuity between the treatment and home systems by allowing parent, therapist, and school personnel to create a commonality of goals and approaches for the youngster. This responsiveness to the needs of the youngster extends through the day and into the night.

Diagnosis

The issue of diagnosis poses another major challenge to successful treatment. A disturbingly high frequency of misdiagnosis of children is noted in the literature (Staff, *Guidepost,* 1987). The after-school program's experience has been that 75% of youngsters entering the program previously diagnosed are rediagnosed (Wirth, 1986). One cannot treat a broken arm by placing a leg in a cast; the need for differential and specific diagnosis in mental health, to be followed by appropriate treatment, is equally crucial.

Fee Scales

The State of California Uniform Method of Determining Ability to Pay (UMDAP) sliding-fee scale is used. It is a sensitive and just scale but not always completely reflective of a family's financial ability. As a result, fees can be adjusted accordingly to meet the needs of families experiencing hardship. Assistance also is offered to parents whose youngsters might be eligible to receive state medical assistance. The fee structure also includes collection of payment from insurance companies. cash fees are also collected from families who are able to pay or part-pay for services.

Funding for the program has constituted an ongoing challenge. Fiscal issues often appear to be without resolution. Needs consistently overshadow resources, and those resources are imperative in the maintenance of any innovative program. Funding has always been only minimally adequate and because competition for public money is stiff, trying to hold unit costs down is a constant chore.

Staff salaries account for 86% of the budget. Although they are competitive on an hourly basis, many positions that optimally should be funded as full-time, in fact, are not. The net result has been an unfortunate limitation in the field of candidates available for hire because the gross annual salaries are barely competitive at the lower end due to fewer workhours per week. Turnover in those positions has also been excessive, with wages most often cited as the cause for resignation. Most staff move on to similar wage levels but with more hours in comparable settings. The costs for rehiring and training, as well as the expense in time to cushion the blows to the morale of the treatment community, are extensive. Yet the opportunities and resources to rectify this problem remain severely limited.

A continuing challenge is to diversify and stabilize funding sources. Funding is secured through the Los Angeles County Department of Mental Health. One-third is California Welfare and Institutions (1983) funding, and the remainder is direct contract funding through the department. Although the budget has increased annually, so, too, has the program service capability. Grants for innovative program additions continue to be submitted as time permits, but, at present, are not a management priority.

The afterschool program is in its sixth year of operation and has experienced its first change in the directorship. It is probable that change will continue to be a dominant theme. In 1988 the program moved from its first site, a converted mortuary, to a "built-to-suit" facility in a nearby community more central to the catchment area.

These changes, in addition to the constant challenges of operating a quality afterschool program, attending to the clinical crises these troubled youngsters continually experience, managing a budget that is not expected to increase for the first time in several years, in spite of increased costs, and maintaining a commitment to an innovative, rather than repetitive program, will underscore the efforts of the year ahead.

REFERENCES

American Psychiatric Association. (1980). *Diagnostic and statistical manual of mental disorders* (3rd ed.). Washington, DC: Author.

California Welfare and Institutions Codes, Sections 5000-9999 (1979).

California Welfare and Institutions Codes, Sections 5000-9999 (1983).

Evangelakis, M. G. (1980). Day treatment. In G. P. Sholevar, R. M. Benson, & B. J. Blinder (Eds.), *Emotional disorders in children and adolescents: Medical and psychological approaches to treatment* (pp. 235–258). New York: Spectrum.

Staff. (1987, March 5). Childhood mental disorders often remain undiagnosed. *Guidepost*, American Association for Counseling and Development.

Sue, S. (1986, February). *Ethnic minorities: Toward the development of effective treatment and responsive service delivery.* Keynote address presented at the Los Angeles County Department of Mental Health Conference on Services to Ethnic Minorities, Los Angeles, CA.

Wirth, B. A. (1986). *Factors affecting discharge and referral outcomes in a child/adolescent day treatment program.* Unpublished manuscript.

III

Appendix

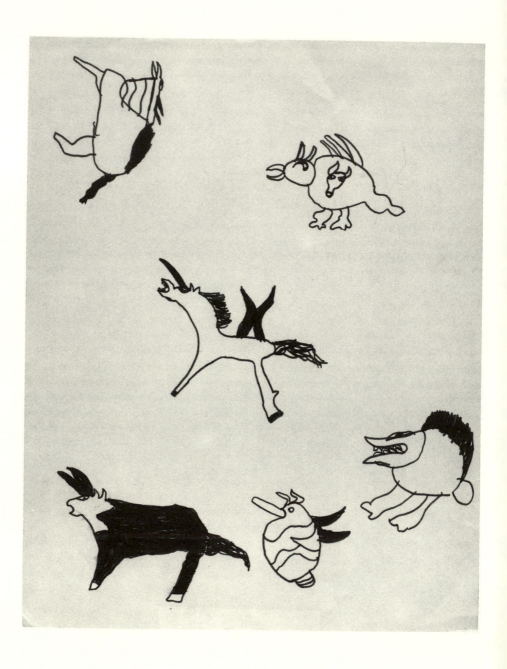

A well-constructed annotated bibliography is an extremely useful source of information. In the editors' many years of work in day treatment, we often sought information about an aspect of day treatment, such as program evaluation, administrative organization, population descriptions, or treatment methods. On several occasions, we found much information and were grateful. On other occasions, we found very little and wrote a review article or designed a system ourselves. Much of the difficulty in finding articles on day psychiatric treatment was due to poor indexing, and searches often required entry into a variety of different data bases. We were eventually surprised to find as many references as we did. Of the 157 references uncovered, 38% were research papers, 50% were descriptions of programs, and 12% dealt with administration issues. In the process of reviewing this large number of articles, Sara Zimet came to the conclusion that an annotated bibliography would serve as an aid to dissemination of information about various aspects of day psychiatric treatment for children. It is offered here as an appendix.

An Annotated Bibliography of Publications on the Day Treatment of Children with Emotional Disorders

SARA GOODMAN ZIMET

INTRODUCTION

The following listing and description of publications on the day treatment of emotionally disturbed preschool- and preadolescent-age children was meant to be as complete as possible. As a result, the many publications included represent a history of the place of this treatment modality in the United States as well as in several other countries. Thus, there was no attempt to critically evaluate papers for inclusion by a predetermined set of criteria other than the age of the children being served.

The organization of the references is alphabetical according to the name of the first author. In addition, in order to assist the reader in quickly identifying the primary focus of a publication, each reference is preceded by one or more of the following superscript notations:

$$* = \text{Program descriptions}$$
$$a = \text{United States}$$

SARA GOODMAN ZIMET • The Day Care Center, Department of Psychiatry, University of Colorado Health Sciences Center, Denver, Colorado 80262.

175

b = Canada
c = England
d = Finland
e = France
f = The Netherlands
g = Norway
h = South Africa
i = Sweden
j = Switzerland
k = Germany
+ = Research
1 = Outcome and/or follow-up
2 = Characteristics of
    child and/or parents
3 = Administrative issues
4 = From Canada
5 = From England
@ = Reviews of the literature
# = Discussions of admini-
    strative issues
^ = Annotated bibliographies

Only when the research was done on programs outside of the United States was the country indicated in the notation.

In those publications where a specific program is described, the name and location of the program is included in the abstract whenever this information was available in the original paper. The reader also may note that summaries of research papers tend to be given in greater detail than those papers in the other categories listed above.

There is a total of 157 references included. Of this number, 91 or 57.9% are focused primarily on describing one or more components of a day treatment program. Fifty-three or 33.8% of the listings are reports of research dealing with program efficacy, specific characteristics of children in day treatment, and/or the prediction of treatment outcome from entry data. The remaining 13 or 8.3% include 6 papers concerned with administrative issues, 5 that review some of the outcome research on day treatment, and 2 that are incomplete annotated listings of the day-treatment literature.

It also may be of interest to the reader to note that the *International Journal of Partial Hospitalization* is approximately 1 year behind in its publishing schedule. For example, papers that were accepted for publication in 1989 are in 1988 journal issues.

BIBLIOGRAPHY

+1 Anderson, D. R., Long, M. A., Leathers, E., Denny, B., & Hilliard, D. (1981). Documentation of change in problem behaviors among anxious and hostile/aggressive children enrolled in a therapeutic preschool program. *Child Psychiatry and Human Development, 11*, 232–240.

Documents changes, over a period of approximately 17 months, in problem behaviors among children between 3 and 6 years old, who were enrolled in a program affiliated with Duke University Medical Center in Durham, North Carolina. Therapeutic aspects of the program included teacher interventions during half-day sessions 5 days each week, with one teacher per group of six children. Children were classified as either manifesting hostile/aggressive behavior ($N = 23$) or anxious behavior ($N = 13$) based on scores from a teacher's behavior checklist completed at the beginning of treatment. Two outcome measures were used: (a) target problem behaviors derived from the entry behavior checklist; and (b) the teacher's behavior checklist completed again at the termination of treatment. The criterion of positive change was change in 50% of all problem areas. The results indicated that (a) 5 children in the hostile/aggressive group showed improvement, whereas 18 did not; (b) 12 children in the anxious group showed improvement, whereas 1 did not; (c) a significantly greater proportion of anxious children showed a reduction in problem behavior compared to hostile/aggressive children. The analysis of change scores by specific problem types showed a clear reduction in problem behaviors across all subjects. The anxious group showed significant change scores on each of the scales; the hostile/aggressive group did not change significantly on either hostile/aggressive or anxious behaviors.

*a Arajarvi, T., & Oranen, A. M. (1983). First contacts with a family whose child is to be admitted to the child psychiatric day ward. *Acta Paedopsychiatrica, 49*, 119–126.

Describes the admission procedure that is used in a Finnish psychiatric day ward for children 9 to 14 years old. The team of the day ward contacts the family before the admission to the hospital for the following objectives: (a) to establish, together with the family, the need for hospital treatment and the family's readiness for it; (b) to collect adequate information about the subject and the family for working out a realistic treatment schedule without delay; (c) to obtain a realistic concept of the subject's natural environment; (d) to help the family to work with its ambivalence so that the members will be able to make a decision; (e) to inform the family of all available details concerning ward treatment; (f) and to make the family members familiar with the ward. Results show that after admission for treatment, the therapy was discontinued in only one case. The contact therapy also yields valuable information about whether the subject should be placed in day or 24-hour treatment on the ward.

*cAsen, K. (1982). A day unit for families. *Journal of Family Therapy, 4,* 345–358.

Describes the treatment programs and techniques used in a family day unit developed by an urban hospital to meet the needs of families and individuals unable to make effective use of medical, social, and other resources. Typical presenting problems for the children of such families include severe developmental delays, intractable school refusal, behavioral or emotional disorders, psychotic or autistic features, and psychosomatic illnesses. Parental symptoms consist of incidents of child abuse, severe obsessions and rituals involving other family members, depression, and/or mild psychotic states. Three categories of families that seem to benefit from treatments utilized by the unit are described: (a) chaotic families, (b) intractable symptom families, and (c) reunion families. All of these family types demonstrate a limited behavioral repertoire and often exhibit rigidity when faced with the prospect of change. They may also feature an inability to establish boundaries between daily life events, generations, sexual roles, and family subsystems. Treatment goals focus on attending to the presenting problems, providing an alternative experience of family life through enhancing individual strengths and communicative capacities, developing parental authority, and helping children to cope with the outside world.

*aAstrachan, M. (1975). The five-day week: An alternate model in residential treatment centers. *Child Welfare, 54,* 21–26.

Describes the Beech Brook program in Cleveland, Ohio, in which latency-aged children spend 5 days a week in full-time residential care and stay with their families on weekends. The reasons for adopting this model were threefold: (a) to support family growth through family therapy; (b) to share parenting between the parents and the child care staff; and (c) to deliver psychoeducational services that provide the lowest intensity of care consistent with improvement sufficient to justify return of the child to his or her family, school, and peer group. The author discusses the philosophy of treatment, the role of the school, and staff reaction to the program.

@Baenen, R. S., Stephens, M. A. P., & Glenwick, D. S. (1986). Outcome in psychoeducational day school programs: A review. *American Journal of Orthopsychiatry, 56,* 263–270.

Reviews 12 studies and discusses the findings in terms of the following dimensions: behavioral, personal construct, academic, social status, family, and follow-up outcomes. Methodological problems and recommendations for future research efforts are considered as well.

+1Baumann, E. H. (1974). The day treatment program. An alternative to institutionalization. *American Journal of Orthopsychiatry, 44,* 200–201.

The efficacy of the day treatment program at Chicago-Read Mental Health Center in Chicago, Illinois, opened in 1965, was examined. Ninety-five percent of the 67 children treated between 1965 and 1971 continued to be maintained at home and in community schools. Only 4 children were in residential treatment, and in two of these cases, such placement was necessitated by the disintegration of the child's family rather than because of ego deficiencies in the child. Results are remarkable in light of the problems presented by the children at time of admission and the fact that many had been considered and referred for future institutional placement.

+[1]Baumann, E. H. (1976). A day treatment program for severely disturbed young children. *Hospital and Community Psychiatry, 27*, 174–179.

Describes, in detail, the Chicago-Read day treatment center in Chicago, Illinois. The program is for young children (2 to 6 years old) who have severe emotional disturbances, often accompanied by profound functional retardation or neurological impairment or both. The primary therapists are child development specialists; most of the treatment is provided in a classroom setting, through small groups. The author reports on a study of 67 young children who had been treated and discharged, including their psychiatric diagnoses and psychological status at intake and discharge, family characteristics, and treatment outcome an average of 2 years and 7 months after discharge. At that time all but 4 of the children were living at home. Fifty-two of them attended public school, most in regular classes, and the rest were in therapeutic day schools.

+[1,4]Beitchman, J. H., Werkerle, C., & Hood, J. (1987). Diagnostic continuity from preschool to middle childhood. *Journal of the American Academy of Child and Adolescent Psychiatry, 26*, 694–699.

Reports on the 5-year diagnostic and symptom outcome of 98 children who attended a therapeutic preschool program at Royal Ottawa Hospital in Canada. Time 1 diagnoses, based on DSM-III criteria, fell into five broad categories: (a) no Axis 1 diagnosis, (b) conduct-type disorders, (c) attention deficit disorder (ADD), (d) emotional disorders, and (e) developmental delay. Results indicated that children with developmental delay or ADD were most likely to receive the same diagnosis at follow-up, whereas conduct-type and neurotic children showed less diagnostic stability.

*[a]Benedek, E. P., & Salguero, R. (1973). A summer day treatment service program. *Journal of the American Academy of Child Psychiatry, 12*, 724–737.

Describes two day treatment programs at the York Woods Center of the Ypsilanti State Hospital, Michigan: (a) a regular 20-chair program begun in 1965, which provided specialized services for those children who could not use the services provided by the community; and (b) a summer program opened in 1970. Both were provided within the context of other services for children. The development of the summer program is discussed in detail. Case examples are provided.

*aBentovim, A., & Lansdown, R. (1973). Day hospitals and centres of disturbed children in the London area. *British Medical Journal, 4,* 536–538.

Day hospitals and centers for disturbed children in the London area are described, and common and individual problems are discussed (the Great Ormand Street Unit, St. Thomas' Day Hospital, the London Hospital Unit, and the Child Guidance Training Centre). Problems associated with day centers, including parents, children, staff, and philosophy of units, are also considered. It is concluded that the day center model can provide a flexible framework for the provision of long periods of face-to-face treatment for reasonably large groups of children, while economizing on the time of highly skilled psychiatric staff.

*jBettschart, W. (1977). Some reflections on therapeutic measures with parents at a child's day hospital. *Acta Paedopsychiatrica, 43,* 23–31.

Attempts made by a therapeutic team (psychiatrist, psychologist, educator, and teacher) to meet the needs of both parent and child in a child's day hospital are outlined. Each member of the therapeutic group relates to each other interpersonally as well as in a coherent psychoanalytically oriented program. Recognition was given to the risk of referring to etiological and pathogenetic theories of mental illness to hide and rationalize libidinal and aggressive attitudes toward parents. It was concluded that the success of therapeutic action does not depend on the methods of intervention only but also on the personal satisfaction of each team member functioning according to his or her professional role (identifying himself or herself concurrently in the common action of the group toward the child and parent). Parental pregenital and anhistorical psychic structures were also discussed with relation to child therapy.

*jBettschart, W., Galland, S., & Brossy, P. (1983). Therapeutic approaches through daily life in a children's day hospital. *Acta Paedopsychiatrica, 49,* 163–169.

The therapeutic activity of educationists and teachers in the everyday life of a day hospital for children aged 4 to 12 is described and analyzed. The dialectical aspect of this approach is stressed, in that the children are offered a space sufficiently protective for their psychic needs and sufficiently challenging in relation to their illness. At the same time, the children should also have enough living space to develop their potentialities for individuation.

+2Blager, F. B. (1978). Response of emotionally disturbed children to auditory discrimination tests in quiet and in noise. *Journal of Auditory Research, 18,* 221–227.

It was hypothesized that emotionally distrubed children would show lower scores than normal children in both quiet and noise conditions on the

Goldman-Fristoe-Woodcock Test of Auditory Discrimination (GFW). Eighteen children between 6 and 13 years old, who were enrolled in the day treatment center at the University of Colorado Health Sciences Center, were the subjects of this study. They were of normal intelligence and had normal hearing levels. The children were individually administered the GFW. The hypothesis was not supported, although the median scores in both conditions for the emotionally disturbed children were lower than for normal children and were within the range of the poor discriminators. Furthermore, one-third of the subjects scored relatively better in noise than in quiet, and a Wilcoxon matched-pairs signed-ranks test demonstrated that this was a significantly larger number than what would occur in the general population ($p < .025$).

+2Blager, F. B., Zimet, S. G., & Farley, G. K. (1983). Auditory discrimination abilities of emotionally disturbed children in day psychiatric treatment: A replication study. *Journal of Auditory Research, 22,* 77–82.

The abilities of 17 emotionally disturbed children between 8 and 13 years old, enrolled in the day psychiatric treatment center at the University of Colorado Health Sciences Center, were studied using the Goldman-Fristoe-Woodcock Test of Auditory Discrimination (GFW), replicating an earlier study and extending it to other factors possibly influencing auditory discrimination abilities. As had been suggested in the earlier study, the hypothesis was tested that there was a subgroup of emotionally disturbed children who would perform better on the GFW when it was administered in the noise versus the quiet condition. This hypothesis was not upheld. It was confirmed, however, that as a group, such children perform less well than the GFW normative sample both in quiet and in noise conditions. Despite normal hearing levels, their performance more closely resembled that of the GFW poor discriminator group. Age, sex, socioeconomic status, severity of disturbance, and intelligence were shown not to be significantly associated with test performance.

*aBlom, G. E. (1966). Psychoeducational aspects of classroom management. *Exceptional Children, 32,* 377–383.

A clinical episode from a day treatment program at the University of Colorado Health Sciences Center is used as an illustration of psychoeducational aspects of classroom management. These aspects include (a) a psychoeducational orientation, (b) classroom structure, (c) teaching and management styles, (d) program planning in general and for specific children, and (e) behavioral management.

*aBlom, G. E. (1972). A psychoanalytic viewpoint of behavior modification in clinical and educational settings. *Journal of the American Academy of Child Psychiatry, 11,* 675–693.

A point of view is presented suggesting the use of behavior modification with children in clinical and educational settings that are viewed as predominantly psychoanalytic in their orientation. Examples of its application in a day treatment center at the University of Colorado Health Sciences Center are given.

#Blom, G. E., & Finzer, W. F. (1962). The development of specific treatment approaches to the emotionally disturbed child: Psychiatric inpatient and day care treatment. *American Journal of the Medical Sciences, 243,* 166–177.

The variety of treatment approaches that is needed to meet the diverse needs of emotionally disturbed children and their parents is discussed, with particular focus on inpatient and day treatment. These latter two treatment modalities are described in terms of their historical development, their costs and characteristics, the extent and needs for such facilities, indications for their use, and the contents of their programs.

+1Blom, G. E., Farley, G. K., & Ekanger, C. (1973). A psychoeducational treatment program: Its characteristics and results. In G. E. Blom & G. K. Farley (Eds.), *Report on Activities of the Day Care Center of the University of Colorado Medical Center to the Commonwealth Foundation* (pp. 65–81). Denver: University of Colorado Medical Center.

Reports on a retrospective follow-up study of the first 50 children treated at The Day Care Center at the University of Colorado Health Sciences Center in Denver, which opened its doors in 1962. Forty-eight families agreed to participate. They were interviewed individually and were asked to complete two checklists, one on symptoms and the other on life events. The children and their families were also rated retrospectively from chart material on the two checklists, and these ratings were compared to the ones obtained during the interview. The results indicated that 90% of the children were functioning well in their schools. The greatest gain was made in social relationships, regardless of IQ. Younger children were more likely to have a better outcome than older children. Degree of parent involvement and length of time in treatment did not distinguish between outcome groups.

*aBlom, G. E., Farley, G. K., & Guthals, C. (1970). The concept of body image and the remediation of body image disorders. *Journal of Learning Disabilities, 3,* 440–447.

The concept of body image is reviewed. Its assessment and treatment are presented. The material is illustrated by a description of a 10-year-old child in the day treatment program at the University of Colorado Health Sciences Center in Denver.

*aBlom, G. E., Rudnick, M., & Searles, J. (1966). Some principles and practices in the psychoeducational treatment of emotionally disturbed children. *Psychology in the Schools, 3,* 30–38.

Discusses four principles that have been developed from the first 2 years of operating the Day Care Center at the University of Colorado Health Sciences Center in Denver: (a) the integration of clinical and educational viewpoints, (b) the adaptation of teaching styles to learning styles of children, (c) the structural design of the classroom, and (d) the evaluation of behavioral and personality change in the child. Clinical vignettes are used to illustrate the points being made.

*ªBlom, G. E., Ekanger, C. A., Parsons, P. C., Prodoehl, M., & Rudnick, M. (1972). A psychoeducational approach to day care treatment. *Journal of the American Academy of Child Psychiatry, 11*, 492–510.

Describes a program (The Day Care Center), established in 1962 at the University of Colorado Health Sciences Center, for children between 6 and 12 years old with social and academic problems. The evolution of the program is discussed in terms of phases of development in which significant changes occurred in relation to staff organization and interaction, attitudes and values, models of viewing child behavior, and theoretical orientations. The psychoeducational approach was the outcome of this evolution. The application of the psychoeducational approach to case selection, the diagnostic process, the treatment program, and to transition, termination, and follow-up is presented.

+[2]Browne, T., Stotsky, B. A., & Eichorn, J. (1977). A selective comparison of psychological, developmental, social, and academic factors among emotionally disturbed children in three treatment settings. *Child Psychiatry and Human Development, 7*, 231–253.

Investigated if there were significant differences among three groups of emotionally disturbed children in Massachusetts: (a) 72 children in private residential schools, (b) 129 children in private day schools, and (c) 309 children in special classes in public schools. The following data were drawn from records on file at the Massachusetts Department of Education: (a) psychiatric diagnosis, (b) IQ, (c) parental separation, (d) geographical location, (e) family income, (f) family social position, (g) assessment of the child's physical well-being, (h) the Rutter Child Behavior Scale, and (i) the Wide Range Achievement Test. The three groups were compared on these variables. The findings indicated that the three groups differed on several dimensions. On the other hand, they contradicted previous assumptions that a continuum extended from public school special classes to private day schools to residential schools in terms of the severity of the emotional problems.

+[1]Bryce, A. K. (1982). The relationship between partial hospitalization and community adjustment following a short-term psychiatric hospitalization. *Dissertation Abstracts International, 43*, 1689A.

Two groups of children were compared: (a) those who received day treatment immediately following a short-term inpatient stay, and (b) those who either did not or may have received some other form of aftercare. There were 26 children in each group. The children were between the ages of 3 and 12 years at the time of hospitalization. None had been diagnosed as psychotic, and none had been recommended for residential care beyond their inpatient stay. Three outcome instruments were used, two completed by the children's parents and one by their teachers. A significant difference between groups was found on one of the two parent measures. No significant differences between groups were found on the teacher measure. Other variables examined included stress level in the child's life, history of family pathology, diagnosis, outpatient and residential treatment beyond hospital or partial hospitalization, and present school situation. None of the variables was found to interact significantly with treatment conditions on the outcome scores.

*aBurroughs, C. H. (1985). Working with families of severely disturbed children in a day treatment setting. *Clinical Social Work Journal, 13*, 129–139.

Examines the use and effectiveness of family therapy techniques, particularly structural and systems techniques, in working with the families of severely disturbed children in a day treatment setting. Six case examples involving 9- to 14-year-old boys and their parents and a segment of an audiotape of one family that demonstrates circular questioning are included. The goal of these approaches is to break limited, stereotypical, and unconscious patterns of behavior, causing subjects to reexperience or restructure them in different ways.

*aCarter, G. L. (1984). A day treatment program for black parents and their preschoolers. *Children Today, 13*, 19–23, 30.

Describes the Minority Day-Treatment Program in the core area of Minneapolis, Minnesota, begun in 1982. It was offered by the Survival Skills Institute, Inc., an organization formed in 1978 to meet the needs of black families in that city. The major purpose of the program is to help parents recognize and remedy conditions that are harmful to their children and themselves.

*aChazin, R. M. (1969). Day treatment of emotionally disturbed children. *Child Welfare, 48*, 212–218.

Presents a rationale for the day treatment of emotionally disturbed children and describes the characteristics of a therapeutic milieu, the effects of this milieu on children, and a general approach toward helping children to use a milieu constructively.

+1Cohen, N. J., Bradley, S., & Kolers, N. (1987). Outcome evaluation of a therapeutic day treatment program for delayed and disturbed preschoolers. *Journal of the American Academy of Child and Adolescent Psychiatry, 26*, 687–693.

Describes some findings of an outcome evaluation of a multifocused day treatment program for delayed and disturbed preschoolers. The sample consisted of 55 children, 3 to 6 years of age, attending a therapeutic preschool, and 45 nonclinical comparison children. A battery of objective developmental, behavioral, and clinical measures was administered at an initial test point, again 8 to 9 months later, and at discharge for children in the therapeutic preschool only. The results indicated that children with developmental delays and associated emotional and behavioral problems made the most gains, particularly those who initially had nonverbal IQ scores within the normal range. Gains were not observed among children who presented primarily with behavior problems. The results also suggest that intervention for delayed children needs to be prolonged and that the time required for gains to be observed depends on the area of functioning being considered and the child's initial developmental level.

*cConnell, P. H. (1961). The day patient approach in child psychiatry. *Journal of Mental Science, 107,* 969–977.

Describes the development in 1957 of a day hospital for children at Tiverlands in Tyneside, England, a community of 1,250,000 people. The advantages of such a treatment approach are discussed as is the relationship with other programs for emotionally disturbed children in the community.

*aCooke, R. M., & Parsons, P. C. (1969). The listening class: An opportunity to advance skills of attending to, concentrating on, and utilizing auditory information in emotionally disturbed children. *Journal of Special Education, 2,* 329–336.

Describes an innovative clinical/teaching intervention with children at the Day Care Center at the University of Colorado Health Sciences Center in Denver. The goals of the Listening Class were (a) to take a reflective attitude toward auditory information, (b) to learn to analyze the complex auditory environment and to be able to break it down into simpler elements, and (c) to organize these elements into a meaningful context. The class met twice a week for 40-minute sessions over the schoolyear. At first, simple sounds made by familiar objects were played, one at a time; the group analyzed each sound to decide what kind of material might make it. Then, increasingly complex sounds and objects were introduced. The children listened to the recordings, raised their hands if they had any clue, and were asked questions to encourage them to examine their own ideas and to build upon previous experiences in trying to identify the material used to make the sounds. When the group had achieved a high level of skill in approaching the task, the next stage of discovery was introduced that utilized the detective model. The children were presented with sound mysteries consisting of sequences of sounds associated with familiar activities. They were expected to figure out what was happening. Vignettes are presented to illustrate the children's responses at each of the stages.

*cCooklin, A., Miller, A. C., & McHugh, B. (1983). An institution for change: Developing a family day unit. *Family Process, 22,* 453–468.

Describes the theory and structure of a day unit at Marlborough Family Service in London, England. The program was designed to intervene in the systems of families who present with severe or multiple problems to agencies attempting to help them but who are difficult to engage in a therapeutic pact and unresponsive to attempts at outpatient therapy. An analysis of these families is offered in terms of the relations between internal and external boundaries and difficulties in making transitions in the daily contexts of life. The principles of the unit are described in terms of the creation of an artificial extended family, the intensification of sequence and patterns of interaction, and the making and traversing of boundaries. Particular attention is paid to the function of agency interventions in family patterns and to redefining the relationship between family and agencies.

+ [1]Corkey, C. L., & Zimet, S. G. (1987). Relationships with family and friends in young adulthood: A follow-up of children treated in a day hospital. *International Journal of Partial Hospitalization, 4,* 97–115.

Interpersonal relationships were investigated in a group of 51 young adults who had been treated in a day psychiatric hospital during their middle childhood years from a developmental object relations perspective. Data were collected from 48.2% of the potential sample during individual, 2-hour, semistructured interviews. Transcripts of interviews were scored using three rating scales: (a) one tapping relationships with parents; (b) the second characterizing relationships with friends; and (c) the third describing the support seen as available from family, significant others, and friends. Comparisons were made with the standardization population on the parent relationship measure. The findings indicated that the majority of young adults were at developmentally appropriate levels in their interpersonal relationships with parents, friends, and significant others. There were more similarities than differences in the comparison between the study sample and the standardization sample. The effects of gender, age, and severity of psychopathology when day treatment began on interpersonal relationships in young adulthood are discussed.

*[a]Critchley, D. L., and Berlin, I. N. (1979). Day treatment of young psychotic children and their parents: Interdisciplinary issues and problems. *Child Psychiatry and Human Development, 9,* 227–237.

Describes the establishment of the Children's Day Treatment Program in Davis, California. It provides an intensive psychotherapeutic and psychoeducational milieu approach to the treatment of young preschool and school-age psychotic children in a community mental health center setting. It was felt that a high level of parent participation in the milieu led to early identification of parental resistances and parent–staff conflicts. Such rapid problem identification and confrontation permitted earlier effective parent–staff collaboration and a more rapid involvement of parents in the treatment process.

*[a]Critchley, D. L., & Berlin, I. N. (1981). Parent participation in milieu treatment of young psychotic children. *American Journal of Orthopsychiatry, 51,* 149–155.

Describes parent involvement in a day treatment program for psychotic children. Develops the thesis that parental participation in the milieu and educational aspects of the program and in family, couple, or individual psychotherapy is critical to the improvement or recovery of the disturbed child. Working with staff helps satisfy parental needs for nurturance and competency. For staff, who often identify with the child, frequent open discussion and supervision are required to facilitate working effectively with both parent and child. A clinical vignette of a 4-year-old male illustrates the process.

+[1]Culp, R. E., Richardson, M. T., & Heide, J. S. (1987). Differential developmental progress of maltreated children in day treatment. *Social Work, 32,* 497–499.

Investigated the developmental progress of 109 maltreated infants and young children (M age = 2.8 years) enrolled in a therapeutic day treatment program. Developmental test scores were analyzed to evaluate the program's differential effects on three subgroups of these children. These subgroups were defined by sex, race, and reason for intake into the program. The findings indicate that different areas of developmental functioning were significantly related to sex and intake characteristics of the children. Children who were enrolled for prevention of maltreatment benefited least from the program.

#Cuyler, R. N., & Galbraith, J. T. (1988). *Insurance and partial hospitalization.* (Available from The American Association for Partial Hospitalization, 1411 K Street NW, Suite 1000, Washington, DC 20009.)

Provides an overview of health insurance, a summary of the current status of partial hospitalization coverage, and some practical information on how providers can work with the system to arrange for partial hospitalization coverage for their patients when it is not offered in their insurance policies. A review of Medicare coverage of partial hospitalization is also included.

+[5]Daws, D. (1983). Resistance and co-operation: The need for both. A further study of psychotherapy in a day unit. *Journal of Child Psychotherapy, 9,* 143–159.

Discusses the psychotherapy of a 6-year-old girl in a psychoanalytically oriented psychiatric day unit attached to a child guidance center in order to illustrate how psychotherapy fits into the institution. Examples of how staff members either cooperated or did not cooperate in the course of the subject's therapy are presented.

*aDingman, P. R. (1964). Day hospitals for children. In R. L. Epps & L. D. Hanes (Eds.), *Day care of psychiatric patients* (pp. 53–65). Springfield, IL: Charles C Thomas.

Describes the variety of day treatment programs and the terminology used for such programs. The author provides guidelines for helping to distinguish between a day school and a day hospital. He also discusses the basic requirements of a therapeutic environment. Finally, the author describes the program operating at the Des Moines Child Guidance Center in Iowa for 6 years.

*ªDingman, P. R. (1969). Day programs for children—A note on terminology. *Mental Hygiene, 53,* 646–647.

In an attempt to distinguish among the growing variety of day treatment facilities for children, definitions of settings are suggested. Towards this end, five ways of describing the distinguishing features of a program are listed.

+²Doan, R. J., & Petti, T. A. (1989). Clinical and demographic characteristics of child and adolescent partial hospitalization patients. *Journal of the American Academy of Child and Adolescent Psychiatry, 28,* 66–69.

Surveyed 18 child and adolescent partial hospital programs in western Pennsylvania through site visits. The demographic and diagnostic characteristics of 796 patients and clinical records of current and discharged patients were examined. The results indicated that (a) the great majority of patients were white (78%) and relatively poor (69%); (b) 85% lived with relatives and 14.6% in foster homes or other residential facilities; (c) girls compromised 23.6% of the patients; (d) only 3.4% were under 6 years old; (d) the most frequent primary diagnosis was conduct disorder (30%); (e) externalizing disorders accounted for 58% of the diagnoses; (f) children were more likely than adolescents to receive an externalizing disorder diagnosis and less likely to be diagnosed as having an affective disorder; (g) girls were less likely than boys to be labeled as having an externalizing disorder; (h) most current patients lived with relatives, and 52% received Medicaid; (i) 58% had a primary diagnosis of an externalizing disorder, and 46% had been hospitalized; and (j) 40% of the former patients were discharged when such services were no longer needed, and another 36% left because of lack of improvement. Other findings include prior and post-mental-health care and sources of referrals.

*ªDrabman, R., Spitalnik, R., Hagamen, M. B., & Van Witsen, B. (1973). The five-two program: An integrated approach to treating severely disturbed children. *Hospital and Community Psychiatry, 24,* 33–36.

Describes an integrated treatment plan at the Sagamore Children's Center in Melville, New York, that combines therapeutic activities conducted by a child's family, a special school, and a hospital. After short-term hospitalization, the child is gradually returned to live with his or her family for several days a week. The parents are taught to conduct an operant conditioning program to modify the child's most troublesome behaviors. The child also may attend a special school in the community where the behavior modification program is continued.

*ªEkanger, C. A., & Westervelt, G. (1967). Contributions of observation in naturalistic settings to clinical and educational practice. *Journal of Special Education, 1,* 207–213.

Describes a program of home visits by social work staff at the day treatment program at the University of Colorado Health Sciences Center.

The information secured through home visits was seen as complementing, clarifying, and sometimes revising pictures previously obtained through visits with clinic staff at the treatment center. Issues regarding resistance of clinicians to visiting the child's home are discussed. A parallel is drawn between clinicians and parents regarding their attitudes toward visiting what each may consider a "strange environment."

*aEvangelakis, M. G. (1974). *A manual for residential and day treatment of children.* Springfield, IL: Charles C Thomas.

Detailed information about the organization, administration, and treatment philosophy of the South Florida Center is presented. Each phase of the center's operations is described. The treatment program is psychodynamically oriented within the traditional medical model. An adjunctive therapies service provides recreation, music, and industrial therapy. An occupational therapist is attached to the school unit of the center.

*cFarley, G. K. (1988). Comments on "An American's perspective of day treatment programs for children in England." *International Journal of Partial Hospitalization, 5,* 45–47.

Comments on the Zimet article appearing in the same journal issue on day treatment programs in Western Europe, edited by Zimet and Farley.

*cFarley, G. K. (1988). Comments on "Day hospitals and centers for children and adolescents in Great Britain." *International Journal of Partial Hospitalization, 5,* 15–17.

Comments on the Hersov article appearing in the same journal issue on day treatment programs in Western Europe, edited by Zimet and Farley.

*eFarley, G. K. (1988). Comments on "An American's perspective of day-treatment programs for children in France." *International Journal of Partial Hospitalization, 5,* 209–211.

Comments on the Zimet article appearing in the same journal issue on day treatment programs in Western Europe, edited by Zimet and Farley.

*eFarley, G. K. (1988). Comments on "French day hospitals for children: An overview." *International Journal of Partial Hospitalization, 5,* 185–187.

Comments on the Lucas and Talan article appearing in the same journal issue on day treatment programs in Western Europe, edited by Zimet and Farley.

*fFarley, G. K. (1988). Comments on "An American's perspective of day-treatment programs for children in The Netherlands." *International Journal of Partial Hospitalization, 5,* 147–149.

Comments on the Zimet article appearing in the same journal issue on day treatment programs in Western Europe, edited by Zimet and Farley.

*fFarley, G. K. (1988). Comments on "The history and current status of child and adolescent psychiatric day-treatment programs in The Netherlands." *International Journal of Partial Hospitalization, 5,* 125–126.

Comments on the Verheij and Sanders-Woudstra article appearing in the same journal issue on day treatment programs in Western Europe, edited by Zimet and Farley.

*gFarley, G. K. (1988). Comments on "An American's perspective of day-treatment programs for children in Norway." *International Journal of Partial Hospitalization, 5,* 109–111.

Comments on the Zimet article appearing in the same journal issue on day treatment programs in Western Europe, edited by Zimet and Farley.

*iFarley, G. K. (1988). Comments on "An American's perspective of day-treatment programs for children in Sweden." *International Journal of Partial Hospitalization, 5,* 165–167.

Comments on the Zimet article appearing in the same journal issue on day treatment programs in Western Europe, edited by Zimet and Farley.

*jFarley, G. K. (1988). Comments on "An American's perspective of day-treatment programs for children in Switzerland." *International Journal of Partial Hospitalization, 5,* 85–87.

Comments on the Zimet article appearing in the same journal issue on day treatment programs in Western Europe, edited by Zimet and Farley.

*jFarley, G. K. (1988). Comments on "The day hospital for children in Zurich, Switzerland and the concept of dialogics." *International Journal of Partial Hospitalization, 5,* 65–66.

Comments on the Herzka article appearing in the same journal issue on day treatment programs in Western Europe, edited by Zimet and Farley.

*aFarley, G. K., & Goddard, L. (1971). A rationale and method for sex education for emotionally disturbed children with learning disorders. *Journal of Special Education, 4,* 445–450.

Describes a course of study about the human body taught to a group of 7- to 12-year-old children enrolled in the day treatment program at the University of Colorado Health Sciences Center. The material was taught by a child psychiatrist and special education teacher together.

+1Farley, G. K., & Zimet, S. G. (1987). Can a five-minute verbal sample predict the response to day psychiatric treatment? *International Journal of Partial Hospitalization, 4,* 189–198.

Reports on the results of an investigation that attempted to predict treatment outcome by the use of the content analysis of 5-minute verbal samples obtained from children when they entered the day treatment program at the University of Colorado Health Sciences Center. The subjects were 62 children with a mean age of 9 years. The following scales were used as predictors: (a) Hope, (b) Human Relations, and (c) Cognitive Impairment. Outcome measures included several scales from a behavior checklist. The results indicated that verbal sample analysis for the aforementioned scales was only a modestly accurate predictor of improvement. The Cognitive Impairment scale was the best predictor, particularly with children with no organic impairment.

[+][1]Farley, G. K., & Zimet, S. G. (1987). *Cortisol excretion of emotionally disturbed children in relation to stress, anxiety, and competence.* Unpublished manuscript. University of Colorado Health Sciences Center, Department of Psychiatry, Denver, Colorado.

Investigated to what extent urinary free cortisol excretion (UFCE) would reflect certain psychological states measured at the time children entered day treatment. UFCE of 15 emotionally disturbed children in day psychiatric treatment at the Day Care Center, University of Colorado Health Sciences Center, was assessed by the radioimmunoassay method under normal (4 days) and mild stress conditions (the first day of the study and on Halloween). Seven urine specimens were collected over 6 consecutive weeks, 2 hours after a 9:00 A.M. voiding. The psychological states and/or traits being investigated were severity of psychopathology, general anxiety, and intellectual competence. In addition, significant life events occurring at the children's home during the 6 weeks of data collection were recorded. There was no significant increase in UFCE levels from week to week for most children. No relationship was found between UFCE levels and any of the measures of psychological states at T1. In addition, there was no significant increase in UFCE levels on the designated stress days or from week to week for most children. A rise in UFCE occurred with the advent of a significant life event for some children but not for others. Surprisingly, significantly lower levels of cortisol were excreted by children who perceived themselves as being low in chronic anxiety and more competent in their academic work. When lean body weight was taken into account, girls showed significantly higher UFCE levels than boys, and older children had higher UFCE levels than younger children. Furthermore, there was no association between teachers' ratings and children's ratings of anxiety or between the two measures of intellectual competence. In effect, UFCE did not appear to be a reliable indicator of the psychological status of a group of children beginning day treatment.

[*][a]Fenichel, C., Freedman, A. M., & Klapper, Z. (1960). A day school for schizophrenic children. *American Journal of Orthopsychiatry, 30,* 130–143.

Describes, in detail, the first 5 years of the League School in Brooklyn, New York, founded in 1953. Fifty children had been admitted. Ten were discharged and 2 withdrawn because of transportation difficulties. Four of the children were discharged after they passed the 12-year age limit. One of the four was placed in a state institution. The other three went to a residential center. Two of the three adjusted well, but the third was placed in a state institution. Three other children at the school were so disrupting to their families that the school recommended institutionalization. Another child was institutionalized because of improper care and a lack of cooperation by parents. Two other children made sufficient progress to be able to live at home and attend a regular private school and both adjusted extremely well to this arrangement.

*aForbes, E., & Maddron, T. (1989). Systems therapy in a day treatment setting. *International Journal of Partial Hospitalization, 5,* 237–250.

Describes the theoretical and structural orientation of a program for children between 3 and 12 years old at the Pacific Child Center in North Bend, Oregon. It is a nonprofit corporation that had contracted its services with the Oregon State Children's Services Division.

+2Fox, M. (1985). Maternal involvement in residential day treatment. *Social Casework, 66,* 350–357.

Investigated the relationship between maternal locus of control and maternal involvement in children's day treatment. Forty-two mothers and their emotionally disturbed children were studied. A measure of locus of control was administered to mothers, and statistical data concerning maternal involvement was collected over a 14-week period by members of six interdisciplinary teams. Correlational data suggest an association between locus of control and maternal involvement. A secondary analysis showed that mothers constituted a heterogeneous group in everything studied except poverty and the adversity to which they were subjected. Locus of control was the only independent variable found to be correlated with involvement. Specifically, the more internal a mother was found to be, the more likely she was to be involved in the treatment of her child; the converse also was found. It is suggested that mothers must be empowered both in their maternal roles and in their interactions with the agency.

*aFreedman, A. M. (1959). Day hospitals for severely disturbed schizophrenic children. *American Journal of Psychiatry, 115,* 893–898.

Presents the limitations of treating schizophrenic children in outpatient and inpatient programs in order to establish a rationale for day treatment programs. The development in 1953 of such a program by parents at The League School in Brooklyn, New York, is described.

*aFreeman, G. G., Goldberg, G., & Sonnega, J. A. (1983). Cooperation between public schools and mental health agencies: A model program. *Social Work in Education, 5,* 178–187.

Describes a day treatment program for severely emotionally impaired children and adolescents that is operated cooperatively by a public school system and a community mental health board. The model offers school social workers a way of supplying more comprehensive services to severely emotionally impaired children as part of a total community responsibility. It also responds positively to the changing roles and patterns of deinstitutionalization and hospital services.

*cFrommer, E. A. (1967). A day hospital for disturbed children. *Nursing Times, 63,* 1296–1297.

Describes a 5-day-a-week unit for emotionally disturbed young children together with their parents. The unit is run by a sister-in-charge and three staff nursery nurses, with regular visits by a pediatrician and clinical psychologist. Treatment includes collective activity, such as games, poems, cooking, painting, and special therapy where indicated. The ultimate goal of such a program is to restore the atmosphere of trust and cooperation between the parent and child.

*cFrommer, E. A. (1983). Support and treatment for psychiatrically disturbed adolescents in a day hospital. *Acta Paedopsychiatrica, 49*, 141–148.

Describes the management of 11- to 16-year-old children and their families in a day hospital service at St. Thomas's Hospital, Department of Child and Family Psychiatry, London, England. The service offers group and individual psychotherapy and schooling, along with medical treatment.

*cFrommer, E. A., & Lond, M. B. (1967). A day hospital for disturbed children under five. *The Lancet, 1*, 377–379.

Describes a day hospital for the treatment of psychiatrically disturbed children under 5 years old, where parents are encouraged to enter the treatment setting together with their child. The program began in London, England, at St. Thomas's Hospital in 1962. Psychiatrists and special therapists are used on a part-time basis. Improvement was observed in 50 of 68 withdrawn, clinging, and regressed children, and in 14 of 30 unmanageable ones. There were 15 treatment failures in the two groups. The others showed some improvement or have continued in treatment. Seven of 11 psychotic children improved to some extent, and 3 others were supported through difficult periods without deterioration. One failed to respond to all efforts. Of the 15 mentally retarded children, 10 showed a surprising degree of improvement, but 6 did not respond satisfactorily.

@Gabel, S., & Finn, M. (1986). Outcome in children's day-treatment programs: Review of the literature and recommendations for future research. *International Journal of Partial Hospitalization, 3*, 261–271.

Reviews the literature on outcome of children served in day treatment facilities. Day treatment appears to be effective in returning children to regular school environments and in delaying or preventing residential treatment. Behavioral, social, and academic gains are more modest. Directions for future research are suggested.

+1Gabel, S., Finn, M., & Ahmad, A. (1988). Day treatment outcome with severely disturbed children. *Journal of the American Academy of Child and Adolescent Psychiatry, 27*, 479–482.

Assessed the outcome of 52 of a potential 56 severely disturbed, mostly black children from an urban area and disorganized home and family environments, who had been treated at the Children's Day Hospital of the New York Hospital, Cornell Medical Center, Westchester Division, White Plains, New York. The children ranged in age from 4 to 12 years old. Charts were reviewed for relevant demographic, diagnostic, and treatment data. Slightly more than half the group was referred to out-of-home residential or inpatient hospitalization on discharge. This placement was associated with preadmission variables of child abuse/maltreatment, parental substance abuse, suicidality, and severe assaultive/destructive behavior.

+2Gaughan, E., & Axelrod, S. (1989). Behavior and achievement relationships with emotionally disturbed children: An applied study. *Psychology in the Schools, 26,* 89–99.

Presents and evaluates an ongoing token economy for emotionally disturbed/behaviorally disordered children 6.9 to 13.2 years old, in a combined partial hospital/special school program. The study attempts to determine whether there was a relationship between "on-task" behavior (including academic work accomplishment) and standardized achievement in a token economy. Despite the fact that the children exhibited a high level of on-task behavior, no relationship was found between on-task behavior and standardized achievement.

*aGold, J. (1967). Child guidance day treatment and the school: A clinic's use of its psycho-educational facility for new programming in the public schools. *American Journal of Orthopsychiatry, 37,* 276–277.

Provides a brief description of a construct developed to ease the reentry of children from day treatment and/or special classes for emotionally disturbed children to regular classes. Such a program was carried out at the Rochester Mental Health Center, Children and Youth Division, in Rochester, New York.

+1Gold, J., & Reisman, J. M. (1970). An outcome study of a day treatment unit school in a community mental health center. *American Journal of Orthopsychiatry, 40,* 286–287.

This study evaluated the outcome of 48 of 50 children discharged from a day treatment unit over a period of 4.5 years. The results indicated that 77% were reentered in public school classes, although the majority of them (70%) still required some special educational program. Sixty-six percent of the sample were described as having less severe symptoms at follow-up. The overall picture of the children that emerged from teacher and parent ratings was a positive one.

+1Goldfarb, W., Goldfarb, N., & Pollack, R. C. (1966). Treatment of childhood schizophrenia: A three-year comparison of day and residential treatment. *Archives of General Psychiatry, 14,* 119–128.

This report compares the clinical progress of two groups of schizophrenic children at the Ittleson Center for Child Research in the Bronx, New York, opened in 1953. One group was treated in residence, whereas the other group was treated in the day center over a 3-year period. Thirteen day treatment children were matched with 13 residential children by sex, age at admission to treatment, neurological diagnosis (organic or nonorganic), and intellectual functioning at admission to treatment. The findings indicate that schizophrenic children who were unscorable on the Wechsler Intelligence Scale for Children (WISC) showed no significant improvement in either day or residential treatment. Among those who were scorable on the WISC, organic children in day treatment showed no difference in progress from organic children in residential treatment. Nonorganic children in residential treatment gave evidence of more improvement than nonorganic children in day treatment. The findings are discussed in terms of the disordering family influence for nonorganic children remaining in the home.

#Goodman, M. (1974). Day treatment: Innovation reconsidered. *Canadian Psychiatric Association Journal, 19,* 93–97.

Describes the development of an innovative day treatment center for children in a traditional mental health clinic in Michigan for the purpose of aiding in the development of these centers in Canada. Problem areas discussed include (a) program components, (b) evolvement of staff roles and functions, (c) interdependence and communication, (d) specific organizational outcomes, and (e) staff readiness. In the development of any new program, a major deterrent to the achievement of objectives is the tendency to compromise over ideals because of staff resistance to risk and change.

*bGrimes, C., Garner, L., & Weiss, D. (1983). A day treatment programme for children of school age. *Canadian Psychology, 24,* 131–134.

Describes the procedures and guidelines used at intake/screening and at discharge/follow-up at the Thistletown Regional Center in Toronto, Ontario, Canada. The goal of the procedures is to engage the family and community in jointly planning on behalf of the child.

*aGritzka, K., Berfelz, K., & Geissmar, R. (1970). An interdisciplinary approach in day treatment of emotionally disturbed children. *Child Welfare, 49,* 468–472.

Describes a program at the Child Psychiatric Day-Care Unit of University Hospital, University of Washington, Seattle, Washington. It was opened in 1962 and treats children in two age groups: 2- to 7-year-olds and 5- to 11-year-olds. The major objectives of treatment are (a) to help the children develop skills and behaviors necessary for placement in a special education class or special school and (b) to increase, through family therapy, the parents' ability to understand and manage their child's problems.

+1Halpern, W. I., Kissel, S., & Gold, J. (1978). Day treatment as an aid to mainstreaming troubled children. *Community Mental Health Journal, 14,* 319–326.

Problem children, who are diverted from public school programming into a private psychoeducational day facility in a community mental health center, are followed up in a 10-year study to determine the rate of return to regular classes. The evidence points to a successful reintegration into public schools for the great majority of students. A philosophy for mainstreaming, which supports the need for proper preparation of children for public school reentry, is basic to effective management.

*aHarris, S. L. (1974). Involving college students and parents in a child care setting: A day school for the child with autistic behaviors. *Child Care Quarterly, 3,* 188–194.

Describes a day treatment program for autistic children at the Child Behavioral Research and Learning Center in New Brunswick, New Jersey. The program is jointly operated by Rutgers University and a private nonprofit school for children with learning disabilities, communications disorders, or behavioral problems of organic etiology. Operant techniques were employed to increase deficient language and social behaviors in seven boys and three girls, 5 to 12 years old. Preliminary results indicate improvement in all children except one. The program employed 60 undergraduates as individual tutors and required regular parent participation in behavior modification workshops. Child care workers may play an important role in training parents to work with their own children, supervising the training of college students, and utilizing such students effectively in the care of deviant children.

*cHersov, L., & Bentovim, A. (1985). In-patient and day-hospital units. In M. Rutter & L. Hersov (Eds.), *Child and adolescent psychiatry: Modern approaches (2nd ed.)* (pp. 766–779). Boston: Blackwell Scientific Publications.

Reviews the history, present status, and thinking about in-patient and day hospital treatment of children and adolescents primarily in England and, to a lesser degree, in the United States. The authors note that hospital treatment of psychiatric disorders in children has evolved steadily since its beginnings, where the objectives were "containment," to its present sophisticated use of "milieu" therapy, embodying psychodynamic and behavioral techniques of management. The advent in England of family units, mother–child units, and day hospital units has increased the range of problems that can be treated and opened the way to direct work with children and their families.

*cHersov, L. (1988). Day hospitals and centers for children and adolescents in Great Britain. *International Journal of Partial Hospitalization, 5,* 3–14.

The history of day hospitals and centers for children and adolescents in Great Britain is reviewed, starting with the inception of the first day hospital in 1961. Since then, different types of day units have developed, which have been influenced by the setting, age of the child, and the child's diagnosis. A range of therapeutic approaches has been used. Although the practice of day treatment in either a day hospital or center for infants, children, and/or adolescents has taken firm root in Great Britain, very few studies have been carried out to evaluate the effectiveness of this treatment approach. Those studies that have been done demonstrate the complex nature of the research and the difficulty in fully understanding the data it produces.

*jHerzka, H. S. (1982). Zurich's day clinic for child and adolescent psychiatry: Setting and possibilities. *International Journal of Partial Hospitalization, 1,* 89–98.

Provides a brief description of a day clinic for psychiatrically disturbed children, opened in 1975 in Zurich, Switzerland. Problems resulting from the interaction of the child, parents, treatment team, and environment are also described and discussed, as are the composition and operation of the treatment teams. Finally, a consideration of the dialogic relationship between education and psychotherapy is presented.

*jHerzka, H. S. (1988). The day hospital for children in Zurich, Switzerland and the concept of dialogics. *International Journal of Partial Hospitalization, 5,* 49–60.

The only day hospital for children and adolescents in the German-speaking part of Switzerland is located in Zurich. It has been operating since 1975 within the philosophical principles of dialogics. In this paper, the author describes, in detail, the concept of dialogics as it relates to the beliefs and practices in carrying out an integrated therapeutic environment for children and their parents.

+[1,2,4]Hunter, D. S., Webster, C. D., Konstantareas, M. M., & Sloman, L. (1982). Ten years later: What becomes of the psychiatrically disturbed child in day treatment. *Journal of Child Care, 1,* 45–57.

Attempted to conduct a follow-up study of 72 children 10 years after they had been discharged from day treatment in Canada. Their ages at follow-up were between 16 and 26 years old. Only 14 subjects could be located and, of these, only 10 agreed to participate. They were interviewed using a semistructured interview schedule. Five of the 14 remembered their stay in the treatment center. Of the 5, 4 had negative memories associated with it. Four of the subjects had involvement with the law, one of whom was facing first-degree murder charges. Three of the 14 had not had continuous contact with psychiatric facilities. The authors believed that present social and vocational adjustment could have been predicted, to some extent, by analysis of key information available at the time of discharge.

+[1,2,4]Hunter, D. S., & Webster, C. D. (1984). Children in day treatment: A four to eight year follow-up. *Journal of Child Care, 2,* 27–40.

Examined the current level of functioning of fifteen 12- to 17-year-old males who had been treated in a Canadian day treatment setting 4 to 8 years previously. Information was obtained through self-report questionnaires and interviews with subjects and their parents. Before these interviews took place, six experienced childcare workers, as well as the first author, examined clinical reports and made predictions about the outcome of the 15 subjects. At follow-up, satisfaction with the program appeared to be quite high and, taken as a whole, subjects had fared reasonably well. Some parents had useful advice to offer professionals interested in helping the families of children in care. The predictive ability for the 6 noninvolved clinicians was rather low, although it was unclear whether this was due to the inherent difficulty of the particular prediction task or to the way that task was structured. As anticipated, the first author's predictions were modestly accurate.

+[1]Hyman, M. H. (1973). Efficacy of day treatment intervention: Comparison of two matched emotionally disturbed kindergarten age groups. *Dissertation Abstracts International, 4,* 31909-A.

Compared the effects of a psychoeducationally oriented program across matched groups of kindergarten-age children, who had been referred for possible enrollment at the Wayne County Children's Center in Detroit, Michigan. The experimental group received treatment, whereas the other group did not. The groups were matched on the basis of age, sex, intelligence, socioeconomic status, and symptom commonality. A 37-item child behavior checklist was completed by teachers to assess adjustment. A statistically significant difference between the groups was found on 6 of the 37 items. The results agree with a body of literature that states that there is a 65% to 75% improvement rate in a group of emotionally disturbed children regardless of a treatment intervention.

+[2]Jackson, A. M., Farley, G. K., Zimet, S. G., & Gottman, J. M. (1979). Optimizing the WISC-R test performance of low- and high-impulsive emotionally disturbed children. *Journal of Learning Disabilities, 12,* 622–625.

The effects are examined of five test administration conditions on the WISC-R test performance of high- and low-impulsive emotionally disturbed children, many of whom were in day psychiatric treatment. In addition to the standard procedure, reward for attention, reward for success, feedback on success and failure, and self-vocalization procedures were tested and compared. Children were randomly assigned to each condition. The findings demonstrate a strong relationship between WISC-R scores and administrative procedures. Conditions that provide knowledge of success and those in which payment is given for desired behaviors were powerful motivators for improving the test performance of emotionally disturbed boys and high-impulsive children. Conversely, emotionally disturbed girls and low-impulsive children performed best when given information on the success of their performance.

+[1]Kaufman, A., Paget, K. D., & Wood, M. M. (1981). Effectiveness of developmental therapy for severely emotionally disturbed children. In F. H. Wood (Ed.), *Perspectives for a new decade: Education's responsibility for se-*

riously disturbed and behaviorally disordered children and youth. Reston, VA: Council for Exceptional Children.

Describes a study aimed at providing validation of the effectiveness of the developmental therapy psychoeducational treatment model. Results showed that children receiving developmental therapy manifested a large and statistically significant reduction in their severe behavior problems as perceived by their parents.

^Kennedy, L. L. (1988). *Bibliography on partial hospitalization.* (Available from The American Association for Partial Hospitalization, 1411 K Street NW, Suite 1000, Washington, D.C. 20009.)

Includes 821 references, 105 of which are concerned with child and/or adolescent partial hospitalization issues. Many important papers regarding child and/or adolescent treatment concerns are not included. The organization of the bibliography is alphabetical by first author's name. It is also possible to locate references by 32 different categories. Each of the categories is listed in the front of the bibliography. The numbers of the references relevant to a category are listed below its name.

*aKiser, L. J., McColgan, E. B., Pruitt, D. B., Ackerman, B. J., & Mosley, J. B. (1984). Child and adolescent day treatment: A descriptive analysis of a model program. *International Journal of Partial Hospitalization, 2,* 263–274.

Since the inception of the University of Tennessee Child and Adolescent Day Treatment Program in 1982, a total of 53 patients has received services. This paper provides a broad overview of the patient population as well as descriptive data accumulated during the first 18 months of operation of the program. Several factors that determined patient eligibility and availability are briefly described. Special attention is given to the following variab' ·s: (a) age, (b) sex, (c) referral source to the program, (d) diagnosis, (e) length of stay in the program, and (f) discharge disposition. Interrelationships among these variables are discussed.

+3Kiser, L. J., Pruitt, D. B., McColgan, E. B., & Ackerman, B. J. (1986). A survey of child and adolescent day-treatment programs: Establishing definitions and standards. *International Journal of Partial Hospitalization, 3,* 247–259.

A survey of 82 programs operating nationally is used to assess the present status of child and adolescent day treatment services. Overwhelming variability in the responses leads the authors to suggest criteria for standards and definitions. Survey results are presented for programming issues, patients, staff, clinical issues, funding, and research, followed by specific recommendations in each area. The authors conclude that without substantial change toward standardization, child and adolescent day treatment programs will continue to struggle in the highly competitive mental health care market.

+3Kiser, L. J., Ackerman, B. J., & Pruitt, D. B. (1987). A comparison of intensive psychiatric services for children and adolescents: Cost of day treatment versus hospitalization. *International Journal of Partial Hospitalization, 4*, 17–27.

This paper focuses on the relative cost difference of treating children and adolescents in a day treatment program versus three inpatient hospital settings. The study finds that the populations in the two settings are similar with regard to demographic and diagnostic characteristics and that day treatment is significantly less costly on a daily basis. A conservative conclusion is that over the course of treatment, partial hospitalization is equal to or less costly than hospitalization.

+²Kiser, L. J., Nunn, W. B., Millsap, P. A., Heston, J. D., McDonald, J. C., Trapp, C. A., & Pruitt, D. B. (1988). Child and adolescent day treatment: Population profile. *International Journal of Partial Hospitalization, 5*, 287–305.

Presents the demographic and clinical data used to define the population of children and adolescents served in a model day treatment program at the University of Tennessee, Memphis, Division of Child and Adolescent Psychiatry. On the day of admission, patients and parents complete a battery of instruments designed to measure reliably characteristics of the patient's system at three levels: individual, parental, and family. The assessment allows for comparisons among self-report, parent/other report, and clinician report measures. Results indicate moderate levels of disturbance, representing a wide variety of childhood disorders and dysfunctions with the families.

*ªLahey, B. B., & Kupfer, D. L. (1978). Partial hospitalization programs for children and adolescents. In R. F. Luber, Jr. (Ed.), *Partial hospitalization: A current perspective*. New York: Plenum Press.

Provides a broad overview of "part-time" treatment programs for children and adolescents in the United States. Discusses the following issues: (a) the advantages of this treatment modality; (b) the range of models that exist; (c) the role of schooling; (d) appropriate clients for part-time treatment; (e) the need for empirical investigations; and (f) other alternatives to full-time residential care.

#LaVietes, R. (1962). The teacher's role in the education of the emotionally disturbed child. *American Journal of Orthopsychiatry, 32*, 854–862.

This paper proposes the idea that the teacher of the emotionally disturbed child must function in a special role that integrates both the traditional role of the teacher and the clinical role of the psychotherapist. In order to accomplish this, joint supervision of the teacher by the educator and the clinician is recommended. Clinical vignettes illustrate the points made. The observations for this paper were made largely at the Godmother's League Day Treatment Center and School for Emotionally Disturbed Children that was affiliated with the Mount Sinai Hospital of New York and the Board of Education of the City of New York.

*ªLaVietes, R. L. (1972). Psychiatry and the school. In A. M. Freedman and H. I. Kaplan (Eds.), *The child: His psychological and cultural development: Vol. 2. The major psychological disorders and their treatment*. New York: Atheneum.

Presents a brief overview of the broad components of day treatment. A rationale, a description of who is appropriate for this modality, and the program's goals also are included.

*ªLaVietes, R. L. (1972). Day treatment. In A. M. Freedman, and H. I. Kaplan (Eds.), *The child: His psychological and cultural development: Vol. 2. The major psychological disorders and their treatment*. New York: Atheneum.

Describes partial hospitalization that provides more therapeutic intervention than a child guidance clinic without removing the child from the home. Establishing the proper milieu is stressed, and types of therapies and education are discussed.

*ªLaVietes, R. L., Hulse, W. C., & Blau, A. (1960). A psychiatric day treatment center and school for young children and their parents. *American Journal of Orthopsychiatry, 30*, 468–482.

Describes, in detail, a 2-year-old psychiatric service for children, The Godmother's League Day Treatment Center and School in New York City, which opened in 1956. Twenty-seven children were admitted. The results of 17 children who had a minimum of 1-year's treatment are tentatively evaluated. The data for each child are presented in tabular form and include age, gender, diagnosis, symptoms, siblings, father's symptoms, mother's symptoms, treatment time, and progress.

+¹LaVietes, R. L., Cohen, R., Reens, R., & Ronall, R. (1965). Day treatment center and school: Seven years experience. *American Journal of Orthopsychiatry, 35*, 160–169.

Describes the program at the Children's Day Treatment Center and School (formerly the Godmother's League School) in New York City, which opened in 1956. Outcome was assessed and described for 38 children who had completed the program. The roles of diagnosis, therapeutic responsiveness, family dynamics, sociocultural factors, and educational potential in treatment outcome are discussed.

+³Leibenluft, E., & Leibenluft, J. D. (1988). Reimbursement for partial hospitalization: A survey and policy implications. *American Journal of Psychiatry, 145*, 1514–1520.

Surveyed a sample of HMOs and public and private payers to obtain information about payment policies. The authors concluded that in the private sector, reimbursement barriers are diminishing but that clinicians frequently must obtain an extracontractual agreement for coverage. Partial hospitalization is particularly attractive to HMOs and others that pay on a capitated basis and can strictly control utilization. A recent clarification of Medicare guidelines may facilitate reimbursement for hospital-based programs, but there remain significant disincentives under the Medicare statute for widespread utilization of this service.

*ªLifshin, J. (1979). Child partial hospitalization: A comprehensive treatment approach for high-risk children. In J. T. Maxey, R. F. Luber, Jr., and P. M. Lefkowitz (Eds.), *Proceedings of the annual meetings of the American Association for Partial Hospitalization.* Boston, Massachusetts, Washington, DC: American Association for Partial Hospitalization.

Describes the 10-year-old program for high-risk inner-city children at the Brookdale Hospital Medical Center/Community Mental Health Center in the Brownville areas of Brooklyn, New York. The program was developed collaboratively with the New York City Board of Education, and special education is an integral part of the treatment. A comprehensive network of services is provided by a multidisciplinary staff with the aim of facilitating the development of internal and external resources of the children and their families.

*ªLillesand, D. B. (1977). A behavioral-psychodynamic approach to day treatment for emotionally disturbed children. *Child Welfare, 41,* 613–619.

Describes a behavioral/psychodynamic model in the day treatment of emotionally disturbed children. The approach utilizes intervention strategies aimed at the home, school, and community systems in which the child is involved before, during, and after the child's enrollment. It illustrates an ecological orientation to children's mental health care. The program is seen as a short-term, low-cost alternative to residential care.

*ᵉLucas, G., & Talan, I. (1988). French day hospitals for children: An overview. *International Journal of Partial Hospitalization, 5,* 185–187.

Over the last 30 years, with the implementation of a catchment-area policy in France, a number of day hospitals have been created to replace full-time hospitalization or other residential programs as a treatment modality for child psychotics. Considered as one treatment possibility among others available in any given geographic area, day hospitals differ tremendously in how they are organized. The approach to treatment, however, has been inspired largely by psychoanalysis. Recently, parents favoring cognitive or behavioral techniques have begun to challenge that position. This paper contains an overview of the general situation in France and presents, in greater detail, methods used at the day hospital of the Rothschild Foundation, located in the thirteenth district of Paris. Longitudinal studies going back to 1973, point to a need for extreme caution in establishing prognoses as progress can occur when least expected. The authors favor a strategy of ongoing support for parents and children, devised on a case by case basis rather than preestablished treatment plans applied according to symptoms.

*ªMarshall, K. A., & Stewart, M. F. (1969). Day treatment as a complementary adjunct to residential treatment. *Child Welfare, 48,* 40–44.

Describes a program for children at the Eastfield Children's Center in Campbell, California. Day treatment was added to other programs for children in 1966. The authors make a distinction between children served in residential versus day treatment, and present a 5-point rationale for day treatment. They also discuss the issues regarding integrating day and residential treatment.

#Metzger, M. (1987). Establishing a data base: The first step in effective management for day-treatment programs for children and adolescents. *International Journal of Partial Hospitalization, 4*, 271–279.

A step-by-step plan for organizing and developing a computerized database in a psychoeducational day treatment program for children and adolescents is described. The plan is purposefully limited and simple in conception so that it can be replicated in free-standing and/or smaller programs, those who might not have the resources available that large institutions tend to have.

#Millsap, P., Brown, E., Kiser, L., & Pruitt, D. (1987). The marketing of partial hospitalization. *International Journal of Partial Hospitalization, 4*, 199–208.

In order to survive as a treatment modality in the present competitive market, the authors present a brief overview of the marketing process, ideas for developing a marketing plan, and several examples of specific marketing strategies for putting partial hospital programs in the forefront of treatment choices. The steps in the marketing process include (a) identifying the current situation and analyzing opportunities, threats, strengths, and weaknesses; (b) identifying objectives; (c) identifying target markets; (d) delineating strategies to meet identified objectives; and (e) developing means to evaluate the effectiveness of marketing strategies.

*eMises, R. (1977). Comments on the treatment of childhood psychosis in a day hospital. *Revue de Neuropsychiatrie Infantile et d'Hygiene Mentale, 25*, 737–745.

Personal observations are made concerning the treatment of childhood psychosis in a day hospital. It is argued that psychotic children can be mixed with other types of severe developmental maladjustment cases within the day hospital and this setting provides a suitable framework for the institution of multidisciplinary action. It is posited that patient treatment is most successful when simple educative actions and the activities of daily life can be combined so that there is no separation between psychotherapy and education. It is concluded that if this is accomplished, then a transition can be made to a more systematized individual psychotherapy.

*aMoore, S. K., & Rumbaut, C. (1985). Innovative group therapy and behavior management techniques with children in a partial-care setting. In J. T.

Maxey (Ed.), *Proceedings of the annual meetings of the American Association for Partial Hospitalization,* Boston, Massachusetts. Washington, DC: American Association for Partial Hospitalization.

Describes the DayGlo Children's Group Treatment Program for elementary-school-aged children that uses the outdoors as a program site. The program has been open for 9 years.

*gNaess, P. O., & Spurkland, I. (1983). Family day treatment for children and adolescents. *Acta Paedopsychiatrica, 49,* 133–140.

Describes two day treatment programs in Oslo. One is for preschool children at the Child Psychiatric Hospital that has been operating since 1977. In this program, one of the child's parents is admitted along with the child. At times, younger siblings have been included. The other program is the Family Day Ward at the Adolescent Clinic, which has been open since 1978. The integration of formal family therapeutic sessions with direct environmental therapeutic intervention is characteristic of both programs.

*aNichtern, S., Donahue, G. T., O'Shea, J., Marans, M., Curtis, M., & Brody, C. (1964). A community educational program for the emotionally disturbed child. *American Journal of Orthopsychiatry, 34,* 705–713.

Describes a special educational program for severely emotionally disturbed children established within the existing school system of a community in Elmont, New York. The children are between 5 and 9 years old and range in psychopathology from withdrawn autistic children to exceedingly aggressive, hostile, disruptive children. The outcomes after 1 year and 6 months are presented for six of the children treated.

@Parker, S., & Knoll, J. L., III. (1990). Partial hospitalization: An update. *American Journal of Psychiatry, 147,* 156–160.

Reviews the definitions, historical development, therapeutic and fiscal advantages, and referral patterns of partial hospitalization. The authors conclude that underutilization of this treatment modality will continue until the following three situations change: (a) psychiatrists are trained in the use of partial hospitalization, (b) more standardization of this treatment modality occurs, and (c) third party payers direct patients and doctors toward partial hospitalization.

+1Prentice-Dunn, S., Wilson, D. R., & Lyman, R. D. (1981). Client factors related to outcome in a residential and day treatment program for children. *Journal of Clinical Child Psychology, 10,* 188–191.

The influence of five preadmission client variables and one treatment variable on behavioral ratings improvement and academic improvement was examined in 50 children 6- to 16-years-old, who were discharged after 1 year from day and inpatient treatment at Brewer-Porch Children's Center, University of Alabama. Structural analyses revealed that the child's IQ, age, parental involvement, and living situation were predictors of behavioral ratings improvement. Parental involvement, race, and IQ were predictors of academic gains. Results are related to existing knowledge of individual client variables' effects on treatment outcome. The research model employed is discussed in terms of its utility for internal program analysis and its contribution to knowledge of intervention effects.

+[1]Purdom, D. W. (1979). A public school comprehensive interdisciplinary day treatment program for preadolescents and adolescents with severe learning and behavioral disturbances. *Dissertation Abstracts International, 40,* 2382B.

Compared two day programs with 20 boys in each, matched for IQ, age, and socioeconomic level. The experimental program, which was sponsored jointly by the school district and county mental health center, was located away from the regular school setting. The children received an individualized psychoeducational program with trained teachers, individual, and/or group counseling from the mental health center personnel, either at the school or agency. Parents were offered either individual and/or group counseling. The control program was carried out in the regular school setting. The children had either a part-time tutor or some classes with teachers in a resource room. All the children were mainstreamed into some academic subject areas with regular classroom teachers. The children ranged in age from preadolescence to adolescence and were identified as having severe learning and behavioral disturbances. Pre- and posttreatment measures were administered. Both groups made substantial progress in the academic areas. However, 17 of the 20 children in the control program received failing grades in the subject areas for which they were mainstreamed. The experimental program subjects made substantial gains regarding their feelings about themselves and others. Parents in the experimental group also acquired more positive feelings about their sons.

+[1,4]Richman, N., Graham, P., & Stevenson, J. (1983). Long-term effects of treatment in a pre-school day centre: A controlled study. *British Journal of Psychiatry, 142,* 71–77.

Describes a 5-year follow-up of 25 children who attended a psychiatric day centre for preschool children at London's Hospital for Sick Children. This group was compared at 8 years of age with two matched control groups who had not received intensive treatment. There were few differences between the treated and untreated groups. Possible reasons for the findings are discussed, and some methodological issues involved in carrying out evaluation studies are raised.

*[h]Robertson, B. A., & Friedberg, S. (1979). Follow-up study of children admitted to a psychiatric day centre. *South African Medical Journal, 56,* 1129–1131.

Describes the Red Cross War Memorial Children's Hospital Day Centre

Program in Capetown, South Africa, which was opened in 1975. Descriptive statistics are presented of the first 20 children treated. The psychiatric status of the children and their families was evaluated at admission, discharge, and follow-up. The results indicate that younger children benefit more than older ones from day hospital treatment and that more attention must be paid to the psychiatric needs of the family as a whole.

+2Rogers, S. J., Lewis, H. C., Pantone, J., & Reis, K. (1986). An approach for enhancing the symbolic, communicative, and interpersonal functioning of young children with autism and severe emotional handicaps. *Journal of the Division of Early Childhood 10,* 135–148.

An intervention approach emphasizing development of symbolic thought, communication, and interpersonal relationships was implemented with 26 children, ages 2 through 6, who had infantile autism, pervasive developmental disorder, or severe emotional handicaps. The main intervention strategy was the use of play in all its interpersonal, cognitive, and structural variety, imbedded in a reactive language environment. Over a 6- to 8-month intervention period, the children demonstrated significant changes in several targeted developmental areas, including cognition, perceptual/fine motor, social/emotional, and language skills. Cognitive complexity of their play skills increased significantly in areas of symbolic complexity, symbolic agent, and symbolic substitutions. Additionally, significant improvement in the communicative and interpersonal characteristics of their play was found. These changes support the efficacy of this approach with young autistic and severely emotionally handicapped children when the children's needs for high levels of structure, intensity, and consistency are met.

+2Rogers, S. J., Lewis, H. C., & Reis, K. (1987). An effective procedure for training early special education teams to implement a model program. *Journal of the Division of Early Childhood, 11,* 180–188.

Assessed the efficacy of a set of procedures developed for training early childhood special education teams to use the Playschool Model for young autistic or severely disturbed, developmentally delayed children in center-based special education preschool classes. Twenty team members serving 11 autistic young children and 10 other developmentally disabled children participated in the training. Data were collected on the trainees and on the target children. Child performance was assessed prior to implementation of the model program and approximately 4 months later. Evaluation of training effects revealed (a) positive subjective perception of the value and utility of the training; (b) significant positive increases in knowledge regarding child development, infantile autism, and the Playschool Model; and (c) significant positive changes in the children in five key developmental domains above and beyond what would have been expected had they continued to receive their regular preschool intervention program. Earlier findings concerning the ability of the Playschool Model program to enhance the development of young autistic children were replicated in this study.

+²Rogers, S. J., & Lewis, H. (1989). An effective day treatment model for young children with pervasive developmental disorders. *Journal of the American Academy of Child and Adolescent Psychiatry, 28,* 207–214.

Investigated the outcome of treatment for 31 children between the ages of 2 and 6 years old with DSM-III diagnoses of infantile autism or pervasive developmental disorder. The children were treated over a 6-month period at the Day Treatment Center in the Department of Psychiatry at the University of Colorado Health Sciences Center in Denver. The main intervention strategies were (a) use of positively charged affective experiences to aid the development of close interpersonal relationships, (b) use of play in all its interpersonal, cognitive, and structural variety, and (c) a pragmatics-based language therapy model delivered within a highly predictable and carefully structured milieu. The children demonstrated significant treatment effects in cognition, perceptual/fine motor skills, and social/emotional and language skills, all of which were maintained or increased over a 12- to 18-month treatment period. Play skills increased significantly in symbolic complexity, symbolic agency, and symbolic substitutions. Additionally, there was significant reduction of autistic symptomology.

*ªRoss, A. L. (1974). Combining behavior modification and group work techniques in a day treatment center. *Child Welfare, 53,* 435–444.

Describes the application of behavior modification techniques to small groups of emotionally disturbed children in a day treatment setting and the maintenance of these changes through a therapeutically planned program. The general format of the group meetings was taken from the Tennessee Re-Education Model. This intervention was carried out at the Bellefaire Residential Treatment Center For Children in Cleveland, Ohio. The author concludes that this approach was both practical and effective in modifying the peer group structure to create a positive peer culture.

*ªRoss, A. L., & Schreiber, L. J. (1975). Bellefaire's day treatment program: An interdisciplinary approach to the emotionally disturbed child. *Child Welfare, 54,* 183–194.

Describes the Bellefaire Child Care program in Cleveland, Ohio, begun 3.5 years earlier for children 7 to 14 years old. It serves children with behavior disorders, neurotic children, children manifesting bizarre behavior, and those with immature personality patterns. In addition to discussing the various components of the program, impressions of the success of each of the various program components are outlined. The authors perceive the program as a very successful one.

+ 1Sack, W. H., Mason, R., & Collins, R. (1987). A long-term follow-up study of a children's psychiatric day treatment center. *Child Psychiatry and Human Development, 18,* 58–68.

Describes a follow-up study of 79 children treated for an average of 18 months at Children's Psychiatric Day Treatment Center in Portland, Oregon. The program began in 1970. The investigation was carried out using interviews with parents and/or caretakers and retrospective chart ratings of pretreatment status, diagnosis, and treatment course. DSM-III diagnostic groupings proved to be the strongest correlate of posttreatment success. Children in the broad category of emotional disorders fared best; those in the psychotic and behaviorally disturbed groups continued to be actively symptomatic and were more frequently in special education or institutional settings. Family stability was also associated with posttreatment success. Children who came from a home characterized by divorce or foster care were more frequently institutionalized or in special education classes. The results also demonstrated the importance of parents' involvement in the child's treatment and the need for ongoing services following discharge.

+ 3Sadler, J. E., & Blom, G. E. (1970). "Standby": A clinical research study of child deviant behavior in a psychoeducational setting. *Journal of Special Education, 4,* 89–103.

Presents a quantitative method of studying a classroom behavior management program, referred to as "Standby," at the Day Care Center, a day treatment program at the University of Colorado Health Sciences Center in Denver. Data were collected on 169 Standby events over a period of 161 days. The information recorded included the day of the week, date, time called, the caller's name, the child's name, the nature of the reason for the call, how it was handled, and the length of the interview. The frequency of standby calls was found to be significantly higher on Mondays and Fridays than on other days of the week. Sixty percent of Standby calls came from the teachers with whom the children spent 87% of their time, and the remaining 40% of Standbys came from other staff members with whom the children spent only 13% of their time. A majority of the Standby events were interactive in nature, involving provocations of the staff (44%) and of other children or the group as a whole (30%). The primary mode of handling Standby was to help the child to quiet down and prepare for reentry to the classroom. On the average, the duration of a Standby episode was less than 20 minutes.

+ 1,2,4Schneider, B. H., & Byrne, B. M. (1987). Individualizing social skills training for behavior-disordered children. *Journal of Consulting and Clinical Psychology, 55,* 444–445.

Compared individualized social skills training (IT *N* = 12) with nonindividualized social skills training (NIT *N* = 12), and wait-list control subjects with no training (WLC *N* = 11). Eighteen children were in day treatment, and 17 were in residential care. Children ranged in age from 7 to 13 years and were randomly assigned to one of the three groups after blocking for initial levels of aggression and withdrawal, based on observations. The Social Skills Training program (SST) used in this study was developed at the University of Ottawa in Ontario, Canada. The program consisted of four skill clusters: (a) social perception, (b) social cognition, (c) coping with conflict, and (d) forming friendships. A procedure was used to screen IT children for the skill cluster each needed, but NIT subjects were randomly assigned to clusters. All sessions were videotaped, and 10% were randomly selected and coded by two independent raters for compliance with the manuals. A combined token reinforcement and response-cost program was used to reinforce participation. In the IT condition, each child attended 18 to 24 sessions; NIT subjects attended 24 sessions. An assessment of cooperative play was carried out after training, using a role-playing test and behavioral observations during morning and afternoon recess. Observations were also done at a 3-month follow-up. Role-play tests indicated that the three groups of children (IT, NIT, and WLC) mastered the content of the training sessions to criterion, 87.5%, 76.8%, and 42.3% of the objectives, respectively. Observations of recess play indicated that the increase in cooperative play after treatment was significantly higher for the individualized training group. The improvement in cooperation was sustained at follow-up. There were no significant differences among groups in observed aggression.

^Sternquist, E. F., Gilmore, J., & Block, B. M. (1988). *Child and adolescent partial hospitalization: An annotated bibliography.* (Available from The American Association for Partial Hospitalization, 1411 K Street NW, Suite 1000, Washington, DC 20009.)

Includes approximately 74 references listed alphabetically by the senior author's surname. In contrast to this, the Kennedy (1988) bibliography lists 105 child and adolescent references. As with the Kennedy review, however, many important papers are not included.

+2Stotsky, B. A., Browne, T. H., & Lister, B. (1987). Differences among emotionally disturbed children in three treatment and school settings: Discriminant function and multiple regression analysis. *Child Psychiatry and Human Development, 17,* 235–241.

Investigated if there were significant differences among the following three groups of emotionally disturbed children in Massachusetts: (a) 72 children in private residential schools, (b) 172 children in private day schools, and (c) 309 children in special classes in public schools. The following variables were selected for analysis by multivariate techniques: (a) 26 items from the Rutter scale, (b) IQ, (c) social class, (d) age, and (e) sex. A discriminant function analysis and multiple regression analysis were employed. The findings indicated that the three treatment settings did not constitute completely distinguishable groups. There were no continua demonstrated from public school special class to private day school to residential school for intelligence, academic achievement, psychiatric diagnosis, and behavioral disturbance. These results supported those of the earlier study by Browne, Stotsky, and Eichorn (1977) on this same population of children.

[+2]Stotsky, B. A., Townes, B. D., Martin, D. C., & Browne, T. (1975). Emotionally disturbed children in special schools: An analysis of ratings of disturbed behavior and perceptual handicaps. *Child Psychiatry and Human Development, 6,* 81–88.

Investigated the relationship between perceptual handicaps and adjustment. The subjects were 573 children who attended private residential and day schools between 1962 and 1971 in Massachusetts. Complete records were found on 397 children. The Rutter Child Behavior Scale was completed for each child as follows: (a) at the time of application to the school; (b) at the time of return home; and (c) at follow-up in 1973. Also, two ratings for each child were obtained from school personnel in the special schools at the time of placement and at discharge. The major reason for placement in schools was found to be antisocial and unacceptable behavior in the classroom and at home. A multiple regression analysis, however, found the perceptual items to be very poor predictors of adjustment. In effect, perceptual handicaps may not have contributed materially to, or been influenced by, the antisocial behavior that was apparent initially and led to the removal of the children from their conventional classroom setting.

[*a]Tovey, R. (1983). The family living model: Five-day treatment in a rural environment. *Child Welfare, 62,* 445–449.

Describes the family living component of a community-based treatment program for 3 to 12-year-olds, the Cascade Child Center in Redmond, Oregon. The organization of the program, training of the Family Living parents, and population served are discussed. Advantages of the program include maintenance of the child in his/her community, the family-type experience provided, continuity between day and residential treatment, and parental involvement in treatment and weekend care.

[*a]Tovey, R., & Morton, J. (1985). Adapting multiple impact therapy for day treatment intake. *Child Welfare, 64,* 421–426.

Describes a shortened version of multiple impact therapy (MIT) used in preintake evaluation at the Cascade Child Center in Redmond, Oregon. In MIT, a team of therapists meets for an extended period of time (5 or more hours) with an entire family or household, both as a total group and one-to-one (a therapist to a family member). The structure of MIT is discussed, and illustrations from practice are given.

[*a]Turner, H. W. (1959). The day hospital concept in the treatment of children's disorders. *Journal of the Iowa State Medical Society, 49,* 247–248.

In 1954, the Des Moines Child Guidance Center in Iowa began the study of a day hospital plan designed to provide the most flexible program that could be integrated with its already existing outpatient program. The building accommodated 16 children for 8 hours each day. These children return to their families or other home situations at the end of the day. It is planned that day hospital care will be provided to between 80 and 100 children annually. A research plan to evaluate outcome of treatment has been designed to include a comparison group. Data will be collected at the time of application for service, upon discharge or completion of treatment, and at a follow-up time 1 year later. The measures to be used are described.

*aVaughan, W. T., Jr., & Davis, F. E. (1963). Day hospital programming in a psychiatric hospital for children. *American Journal of Orthopsychiatry, 33,* 542–544.

Describes the development of two day programs for children at Metropolitan State Hospital in Waltham, Massachusetts, in 1958 and 1959, one for schizophrenic children and one for nonschizophrenic children. The authors outline the essential elements required in the development of these services.

*fVerheij, F., & Sanders-Woudstra, J. A. R. (1983). Child-psychiatric day care treatment and the family with pathologically symbiotic relations. *Acta Paedopsychiatrica, 49,* 149–161.

Discusses the treatment of a child from a family with pathologically symbiotic relations, at a day unit of Sophia Children's Hospital in Rotterdam, The Netherlands. In the authors' view, parent counseling is of crucial importance in ensuring the continuation of treatment for a sufficiently long period of time (1 or more years). The professional characteristics needed by the counselor who is working with these parents and the pitfalls awaiting the parent counselor are presented.

*fVerheij, F., & Sanders-Woudstra, J. A. R. (1988). The history and current status of child and adolescent psychiatric day treatment programs in The Netherlands. *International Journal of Partial Hospitalization, 5,* 113–124.

Although its history is a short one, day treatment is in great demand, and an increase in the number of centers throughout the country has been planned. It serves both as a primary and secondary treatment modality. Although the theoretical frames of reference among day units vary, psychoanalytic and systems thinking are the leading orientations. All day units operate with multidisciplinary staff who work intensively and therapeutically with the children and their families. The day unit at Sophia Children's Hospital in Rotterdam is described as an example of an existing program.

*aWasserman, T., & Adamany, N. (1976). Day treatment and public schools: An approach to mainstreaming. *Child Welfare, 55,* 117–124.

Describes, in detail, the behavioral techniques used in a part-time therapeutic day program (The Astor Day Treatment Center) started in 1974 in The Bronx, New York. It was designed to keep children with behavioral and learning disturbances in regular classrooms for part of the schoolday and in the day treatment program for the rest of the day. The goal was to return the child to the school program full-time. Presents descriptive data on 25 children who began treatment when the center opened.

*aWasserman, T. H. (1977). Negative reinforcement to alter disruptive behavior of an adolescent in a day treatment setting. *Journal of Behavior Therapy and Experimental Psychiatry, 8,* 315–317.

Describes the treatment of disruptive behavior in a 12-year-old male in a day treatment program (by negative reinforcement procedure). The use of a negative reinforcer was necessitated by the unavailability of effective positive reinforcers.

*aWeaver, B. J. (1984). Mothers and children: Together, a partial hospitalization program for mothers and children. In J. T. Maxey (Ed.), *Proceedings of the annual meetings of the American Association for Partial Hospitalization,* Boston, Massachusetts. Washington, DC: American Association for Partial Hospitalization, Inc.

Describes a program designed to meet the needs of female clients with children between the ages of 2 and 4 years old, who want to improve their skills as mothers but have limited resources. The program is said to be a cost-effective one.

@Westman, J. C. (1979). Psychiatric day treatment. In J. D. Noshpitz & S. I. Harrison (Eds.), *Basic handbook of child psychiatry: Therapeutic interventions, Vol. 3.* New York: Basic Books.

Provides a historical perspective and a rationale for the day treatment modality for children. The treatment components also are described. In addition, a brief review of outcome studies of a variety of programs is included. Further evaluation studies are called for in order to make clear who is best suited for day treatment and to assess its effectiveness.

*aWhittaker, J. K. (1975). The ecology of child treatment: A developmental/educational approach to the therapeutic milieu. *Journal of Autism and Childhood Schizophrenia, 5,* 223–237.

The author attempts to accomplish the following three aims: (a) identify the major assumptions on which any future model of residential or day treatment for children should be based; (b) identify the distinguishing characteristics of the child population at risk; and (c) identify the essential features of a developmental/educational paradigm of a therapeutic milieu.

+1Winsberg, B. G., Bialer, I., Kupietz, S., Botti, E., & Balka, E. B. (1980). Home vs. hospital care of children with behavior disorders: A controlled investigation. *Archives of General Psychiatry, 37,* 413–418.

Reports on a study that compared community and hospital care of children with severe behavior disorders. The community program emphasized social services and pharmacotherapy. The inpatient program (Kings County Hospital, Brooklyn, New York) included psychotherapy, pharmacotherapy, milieu therapy, and schooling. Pretreatment and outcome measures were collected. The findings showed that community care was effective with regard to behavior control and that both treatments were comparable concerning educational achievement, parent role function, family adjustment, and parent satisfaction with treatment. It was noted that many severely disturbed children who are in dire socioeconomic predicaments can be maintained in the community with special care and intervention. Descriptive follow-up data were collected 1.5 and 3 years after termination and reported.

+ [1,5] Woollacott, S., Graham, P., & Stevenson, J. (1978). A controlled evaluation of the therapeutic effectiveness of a psychiatric day centre for preschool children. *British Journal of Psychiatry, 132,* 349–355.

The progress over 1 year of 25 children aged 2.5 to 3.5 years attending a psychiatric day center was compared with that of 25 similarly disturbed 3-year-old children identified in a total population study. There were few differences in outcome and those that were found did not particularly favor either group. Implications for the organization of treatment services are discussed in terms of the need to lay down clear objectives and to pursue systematic controlled evaluations.

+ [1,4] Wright, H. H., Batey, S. R., Butterfield, P. T., Motes, D. W., & Chestnut, E. C. (1986). Patterns of prescribing psychoactive medication for school age children in a psychiatric day treatment program. *Psychiatric Journal of the University of Ottawa, 2,* 93–96.

Investigates retrospectively the psychoactive medications used in a program at the University of South Carolina School of Medicine. There were 91 children 5 to 12 years old, whose charts were reviewed. They had been in treatment during the years 1970 and 1984. The number and percentage of psychoactive medications prescribed for each child prior to and during treatment were examined with regard to gender, age, and final diagnosis. The differences in the use of medications prior to and during treatment were statistically significant. There were also changes in the use of specific categories of psychoactive medications over the three 5-year intervals in the 15-year period covered by this study.

*[a] Yahalom, I., & Kreiman, J. S. (1965). *Challenge and response: The story of a day treatment center.* Chicago: Jewish Children's Bureau.

Describes the Mary Lawrence Chapter Day Treatment Center for severely disturbed children and their parents. The center serves children between 4 and 8 years old, whose parents are living together and give evidence of a total commitment to the center's therapeutic program.

*[a] Zibelman, R., & Gannone, L. (1984). Attempting to reach the inner-city child: A Kohutian-based partial hospitalization program. In J. T. Maxey

(Ed.), *Proceedings of the annual meetings of the American Association for Partial Hospitalization*, Boston, Massachusetts. Washington, DC: The American Association for Partial Hospitalization.

Describes a program in Philadelphia, Pennsylvania, for innercity children that is based on the theoretical framework of Heinz Kohut. The program is school-based and treats 200 innercity children. Therapeutic sessions are geared to understanding idealizing and mirroring transferences that the child creates unconsciously. The authors report that the process of repairing of the self has led to symptom relief. Two of the main problems discussed include the liaison with school faculties and family resistance.

*a,c,e,f,g,i,jZimet, S. G. (1987). Child partial hospitalization: World view and status. *International Journal of Partial Hospitalization, 4* 243–256.

In this keynote address at the 1988 annual meetings of the American Association for Partial Hospitalization, the author presents an overview of the status of child partial hospitalization in the United States and in six Western European countries: England, France, The Netherlands, Norway, Sweden, and Switzerland. Based on the overview, she discusses six issues related to the future of day treatment in the United States.

*c,e,f,g,i,jZimet, S. G. (1987). *Part 1: Day psychiatric treatment for emotionally handicapped children in Norway, Sweden, and The Netherlands.* (Available from The World Rehabilitation Fund, Inc., International Exchange of Experts and Information in Rehabilitation, 400 East 34th Street, New York, New York.)

In an attempt to fill the knowledge gap regarding day treatment centers abroad, the author visited a representative sample of centers in six Western European countries. The three countries mentioned in the title are presented in Part 1 of her report. Part 2, listed later, includes descriptions of programs in England, France, and Switzerland. Her visit was supported, in part, by a fellowship from the World Rehabilitation Fund's International Exchange of Experts and Information in Rehabilitation.

*c,e,jZimet, S. G. (1988). Part 2: Day psychiatric treatment for emotionally handicapped children in England, France, and Switzerland. (Available from The World Rehabilitation Fund, Inc., International Exchange of Experts and Information in Rehabilitation, 400 East 34th Street, New York, New York.) See previous review regarding Part 1.

*cZimet, S. G. (1988). An American's perspective of day-treatment programs for children in England. *International Journal of Partial Hospitalization, 5,* 19–43.

Day treatment programs for children in England are described from the perspective of the author during her fellowship year under the auspices of the World Rehabilitation Fund, Inc. The day units visited were located in a wide variety of settings including wards of general and children's hospitals, refurbished houses, and public buildings. Some were administered by departments of pediatrics and psychiatry, some by private psychiatric clinics, and others jointly by a public and private agency. Several offered services to children under 5 years old with their parents and others to children between 5 and 12 years old. In the early years, most day treatment programs were based on psychoanalytic theory. Today, however, there is a wide range of practice based on a variety of theoretical orientations. The detailed descriptions provided of the seven centers visited may help the reader to appreciate the range of work being carried out in the Greater London area.

*eZimet, S. G. (1988). An American's perspective of day-treatment programs for children in France. *International Journal of Partial Hospitalization, 5,* 189–208.

Day treatment programs for children in France are described from the perspective of the author during her fellowship year under the auspices of the World Rehabilitation Fund, Inc. Day treatment is a well-established and well-integrated form of treatment in France. It may include full-time enrollment in the center, part-time enrollment in the center and in a mainstreamed community school, or several variations on these schedules within and among programs. Hospital-based, neighborhood- and community-based programs, and privately sponsored programs are described first in terms of the common elements among them and then in terms of the way each program visited is carried out.

*fZimet, S. G. (1988). An American's perspective of day-treatment programs for children in The Netherlands. *International Journal of Partial Hospitalization, 5,* 127–146.

Day treatment programs for children in The Netherlands are described from the perspective of the author during her fellowship year under the auspices of the World Rehabilitation Fund, Inc. It is a relatively new service being provided by both the public and private sectors in hospitals and in community-based centers. Clear distinctions are made, in general, between the three treatment components in which the children are involved: (a) the milieu or life group, (b) the school, and (c) the other therapies. In some units, the child's family is also kept out of these areas, with their therapist providing the links among the various components. In other centers, however, parents are included as observers and/or participants. Systemic family therapy is the preferred intervention with parents. Details of the programs visited are provided.

*gZimet, S. G. (1988). An American's perspective of day-treatment programs for children in Norway. *International Journal of Partial Hospitalization, 5,* 89–108.

Day treatment programs for children in Norway are described from the perspective of the author during her fellowship year under the auspices of the World Rehabilitation Fund, Inc. They are provided through a network of state and county clinics under a national comprehensive health care program. The demand for these services far exceeds the resources available. Possibly as a result of this imbalance, there is a strong movement away from treating the individual only, to a more systems-oriented approach that incorporates a variety of theoretical positions. The programs consist of three elements: (a) the milieu, (b) the school, and (c) a variety of different therapeutic interventions. A full description of the programs visited is provided.

*[i]Zimet, S. G. (1988). An American's perspective of day-treatment programs for children in Sweden. *International Journal of Partial Hospitalization, 5,* 151–163.

Day treatment programs for children in Sweden are described from the perspective of the author during her fellowship year under the auspices of the World Rehabilitation Fund, Inc. It was not until the early 1980s that a major shift occurred from a centralized institutional system of care to a more humane, community-based one. The growth and development of day treatment coincided with this shift. Most child treatment is seen as occurring within carefully planned environments. Thus children may be placed in more than one therapeutic setting at the same time. Details of the programs at each of the centers visited are presented.

*[j]Zimet, S. G. (1988). An American's perspective of day-treatment programs for children in Switzerland. *International Journal of Partial Hospitalization, 5,* 67–83.

Day treatment programs for children in Switzerland are described from the perspective of the author during her fellowship year under the auspices of the World Rehabilitation Fund, Inc. They are not widespread in Switzerland. There is one in the German-speaking sector, several in the French-speaking sector, and none in the remaining sectors of the country. Although there was much that was similar among the centers visited, there were subtle differences that seem to be related to two factors: (a) the autonomy among the three governmental units (e.g., the federal, cantonal, and communal), and (b) the language and cultural differences within and between the sectors. Each of the centers visited is described in detail.

+[2]Zimet, S. G., & Farley, G. K. (1984). The self-concepts of children entering day psychiatric treatment. *Child Psychiatry and Human Development, 15,* 142–150.

The self-concepts of 68 school-age children beginning day treatment at The Day Care Center of the University of Colorado Health Sciences Center were described and compared with groups of normal and clinic-referred children studied by others. The expectation that day treatment children would have significantly lower self-concept scores than normal and clinic-referred children was not met. In fact, a trend in the opposite direction emerged. Seventy-five percent of children beginning day treatment expressed primarily positive views about how they valued themselves. Those with psychoneurotic disorders had significantly higher self-concept scores than did those with personality disorders, and a modest but significant inverse relationship was found between self-concept and severity of disturbance. Social class was significantly related to ratings of self-worth and accounted for 42 percent of the variance. Sex, race, and IQ did not influence self-concept ratings. Treatment implications, measurement issues, and suggestions for future research are discussed.

@Zimet, S. G., & Farley, G. K. (1985). Day treatment for children in the United States: Review article. *Journal of the American Academy of Child Psychiatry, 24,* 732–738.

This paper describes the general philosophy and characteristics of day treatment settings and provides a summary of the research examining their efficacy. The authors concluded that although there appear to be good reasons for the continuing interest in the utilization of day treatment for seriously troubled and troubling children, there is still much to be learned about this population and treatment modality.

+2Zimet, S. G., & Farley, G. K. (1986). Four perspectives on the competence and self-esteem of emotionally disturbed children beginning day treatment. *Journal of the American Academy of Child Psychiatry, 25,* 76–83.

Competence and self-esteem ratings of 34 children beginning day treatment at the Day Care Center of the University of Colorado Health Sciences Center were compared with ratings by their parents, psychotherapists, and teachers. Children's scores were the highest, and teachers' were the lowest. Adult raters' scores showed either a strong trend or a significant difference from children's scores on almost all subscales. There were no differences between adult rater pairs. The results are discussed in terms of the amount of communication among rater groups, the role each adult rater has with the child, and the implications regarding treatment.

+2Zimet, S. G., & Farley, G. K. (1987). How do emotionally disturbed children report their competencies and self-worth? *Journal of the American Academy of Child and Adolescent Psychiatry, 26,* 33–38.

Responses of 68 children starting day psychiatric treatment (DPT) at The Day Care Center of the University of Colorado Health Sciences Center on the Piers-Harris Children's Self-Concept Scale were compared with a similar group of 34 children on the Perceived Competence Scale for Children (PCSC), a measure designed to reduce a socially desirable response set. Comparisons also were made with the PCSC's normative sample. Both self-concept measures drew primarily positive answers from DPT children who were impaired in many domains. They also saw themselves as significantly more skilled at athletics and as varying less across abilities than normal children. None of the demographic variables was related to self-concept ratings. Possible explanations for these findings and directions for future research are discussed.

+3Zimet, S. G., Farley, G. K., & Avitable, N. (1987). Establishing a comprehensive data base in a day-treatment program for children. *International Journal of Partial Hospitalization, 4*, 1–15.

The nuts and bolts of establishing a database for a children's day psychiatric treatment center are described and discussed. Special attention is given to both human and technical factors by providing examples drawn from the experience of setting one up and from clinical data. Illustrations are also included that outline the concepts presented.

+[1]Zimet, S. G., Farley, G. K., & Dahlem, N. W. (1984). Behavior ratings of children in community schools and in day treatment. *International Journal of Partial Hospitalization, 2*, 199–208.

In order to determine the reliability of changes found in school behavior ratings at posttreatment follow-ups, the stability of behavior ratings of emotionally disturbed children by community-based teachers and day treatment teachers was studied when treatment was initiated. This methodological problem was investigated using a test–retest paradigm. Each of 49 children referred for day treatment to The Day Care Center at the University of Colorado Health Sciences Center was rated on the same standardized school behavior checklist by two teachers, one from their community classroom at the time of referral to day treatment and one from the day treatment classroom that accepted them 6 weeks later. No significant differences in mean scale scores were found between the two teacher groups, and all correlations between rater pairs on the same subscales were significant, except for one subscale. Both teacher groups showed similar ratings by child's age and sex. The stability of these findings suggests that school behavior ratings across teachers with very different frames of reference and from very different classroom settings will provide an acceptable index of behavior change at posttreatment follow-ups.

+[2]Zimet, S. G., Farley, G. K., & Dahlem, N. W. (1985). An abbreviated form of the WISC-R for use with emotionally disturbed children. *Psychology in the Schools, 22*, 19–22.

Reports on the results of a study of the efficacy of two multiple-regression-derived, selected-subtest short forms of the WISC-R with children beginning day treatment at The Day Care Center, University of Colorado Health Sciences Center. No significant differences were found between the mean IQ scale scores of either of the short forms and the FSIQ. Correlation coefficients were highly significant, ranging from .958 to .997. Furthermore, only one child shifted IQ classifications when using the short forms. Thus both short-form models provided time-saving estimates of the general intellectual performance of these children.

+[1,2]Zimet, S. G., Farley, G. K., Silver, J., Hebert, F. B., Robb, E. D., Ekanger, C., & Smith, D. (1980). Behavior and personality changes in emotionally disturbed children enrolled in a psychoeducational day treatment center. *Journal of the American Academy of Child Psychiatry, 19*, 240–256.

Data describing personality and behavior characteristics of emotionally disturbed children between 7 and 11 years old during and following treatment in a psychoeducational day treatment center (The Day Care Center) at the University of Colorado Health Sciences Center are presented. Positive changes in social interactions, academic performance, intellectual performance, and self-esteem were documented after approximately 2 years of day treatment. These gains were, for the most part, maintained at the first follow-up 3 to 6 months following discharge and 18 to 24 months following discharge, respectively. The discussion focuses on the process of change over time and on the interrelationships of the changes that occurred.

*[j,k]Zulauf, U., & Herzka, H. S. (1988). Day-hospital programs for children and adolescents in eight West German cities and in Zurich, Switzerland. *International Journal of Partial Hospitalization, 5,* 61–64.

The information presented in this paper was the outgrowth of a symposium held in Dusseldorf, Germany, in 1985. This gathering of professionals involved in day psychiatric treatment of children and adolescents from German-speaking areas represented a first step in a "getting-to-know-you" process. The data collated from the meetings are presented briefly in both tabular and narrative form and include a description of the history and current status of day hospital treatment as a therapeutic modality in Berlin, Dortmund, Dusseldorf, Kassel, Cologne, Mannheim, Marburg, Munich, and Zurich.

Index

221